PICTURE BOOK OF
CHRISTMAS

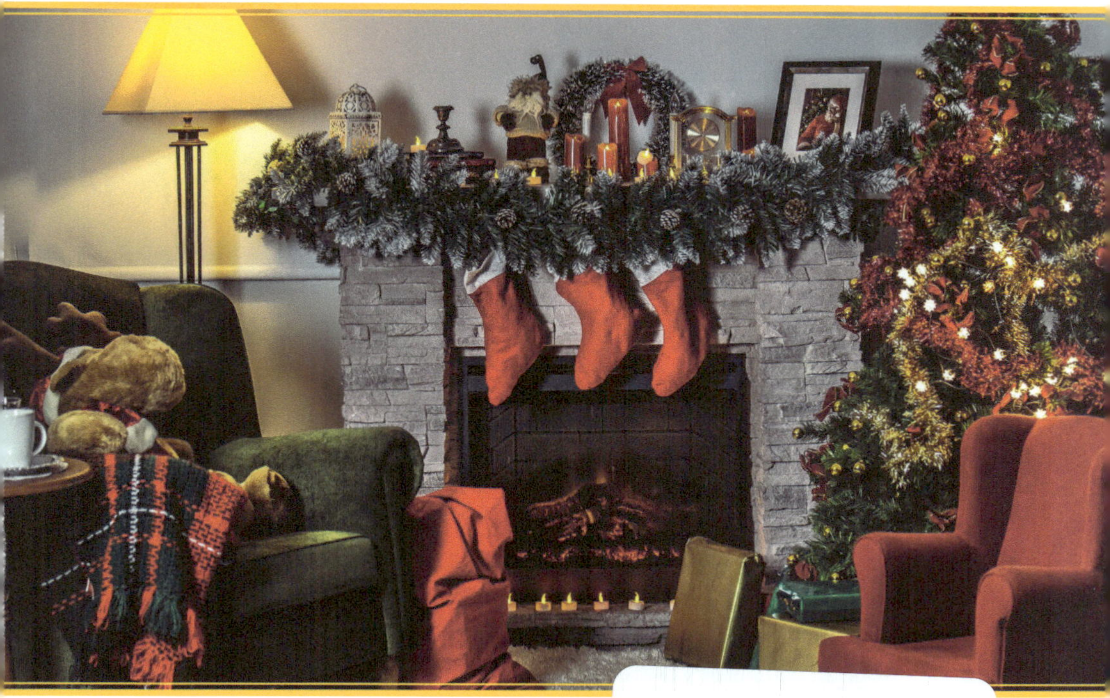

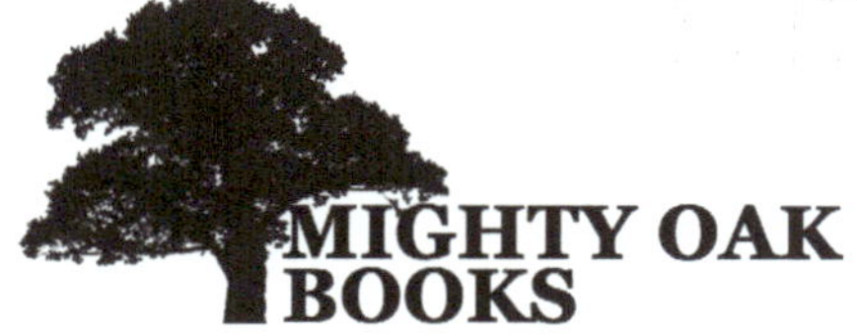

Christmas Angel

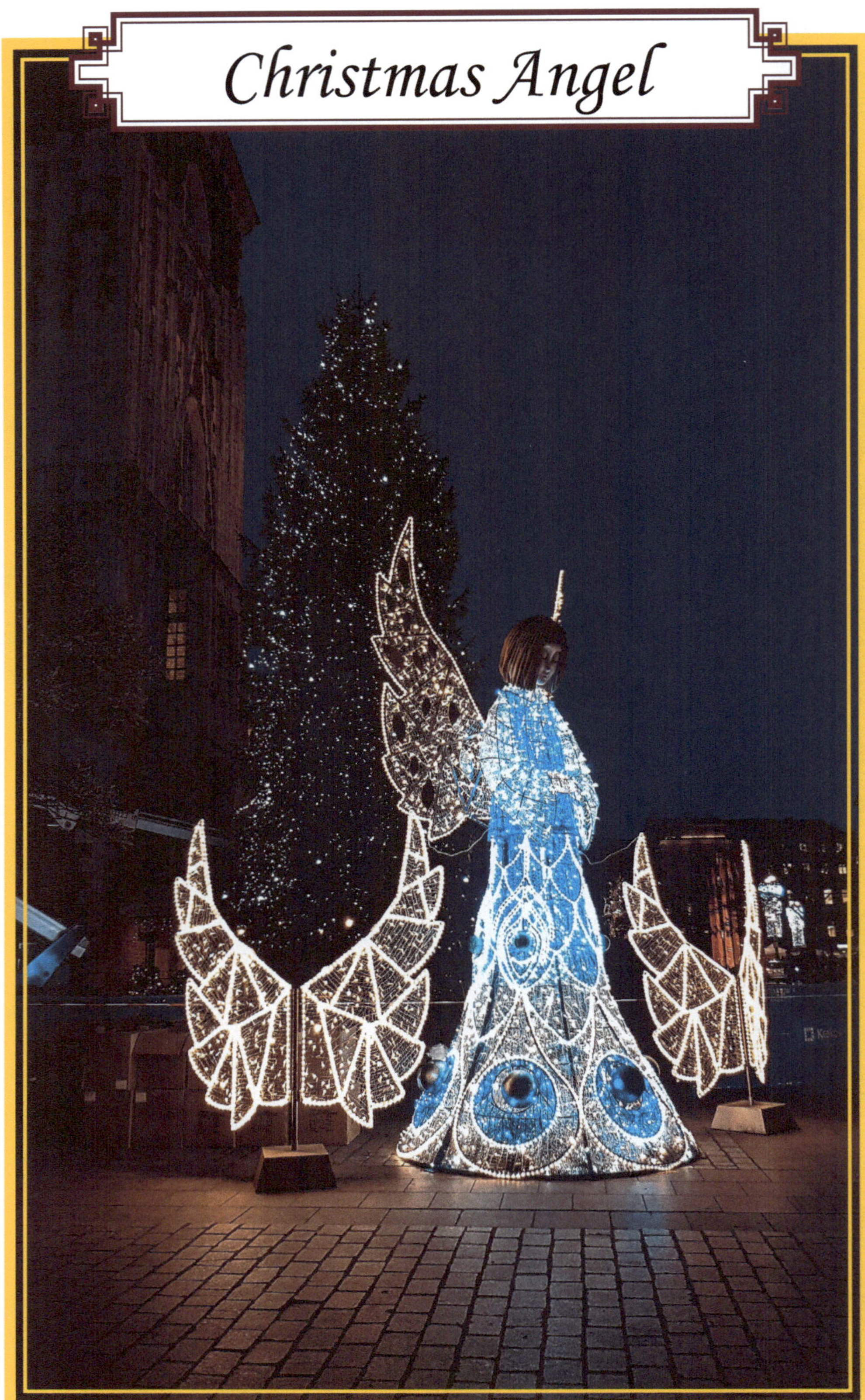

Santa Snow Globe

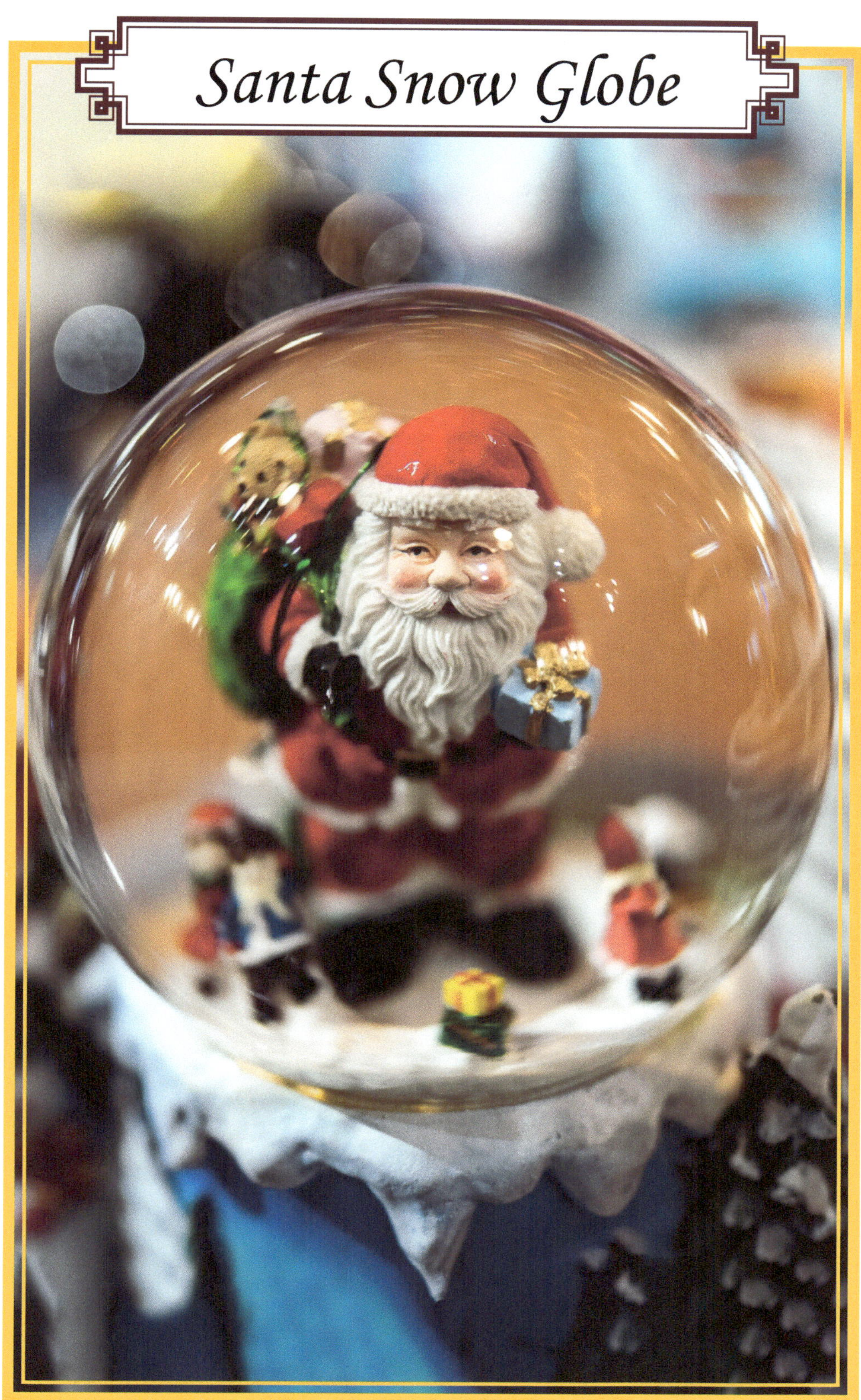

A Warm Drink

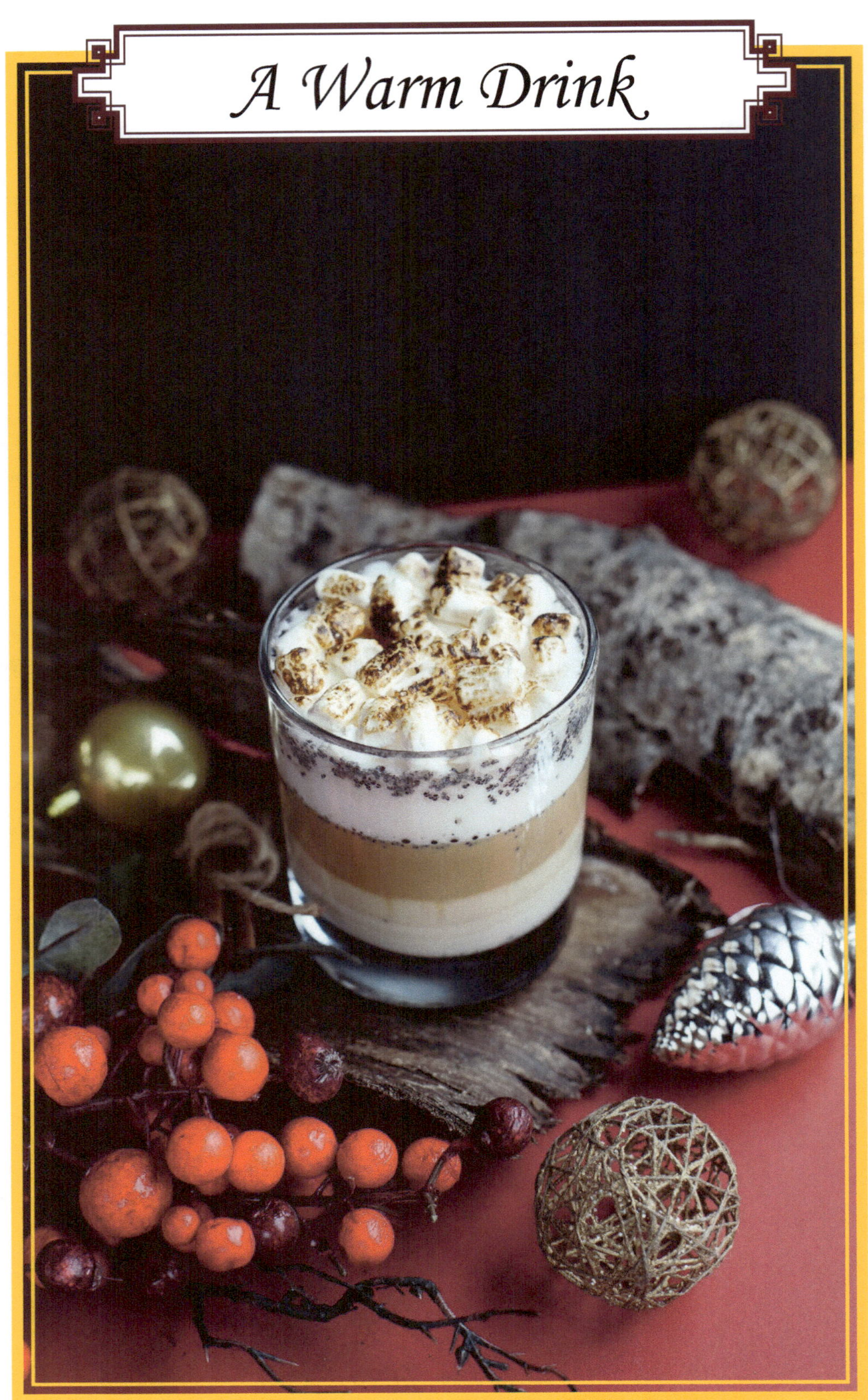

Winter Wonderland

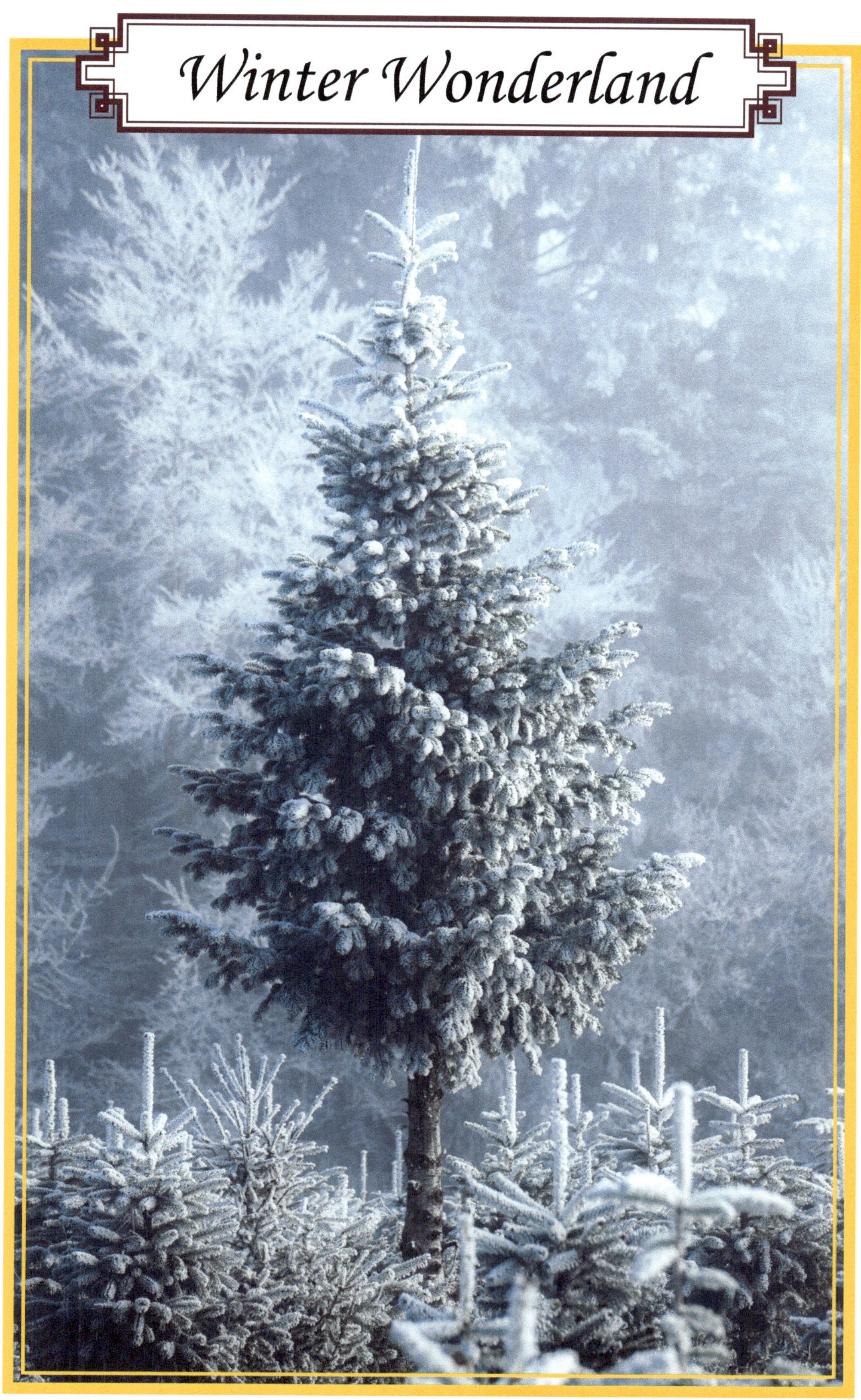

Christmas Wreath

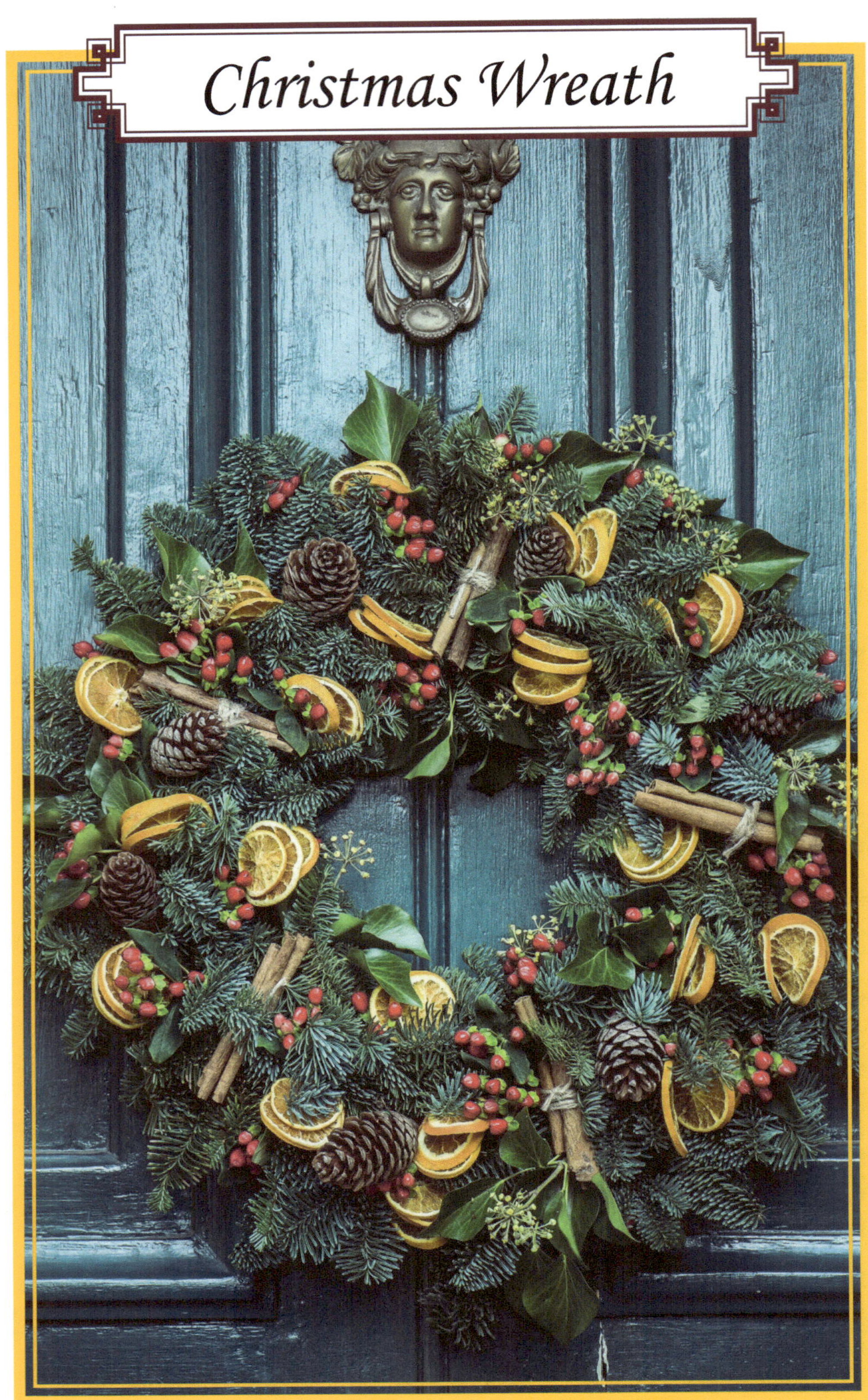

Toy Soldier

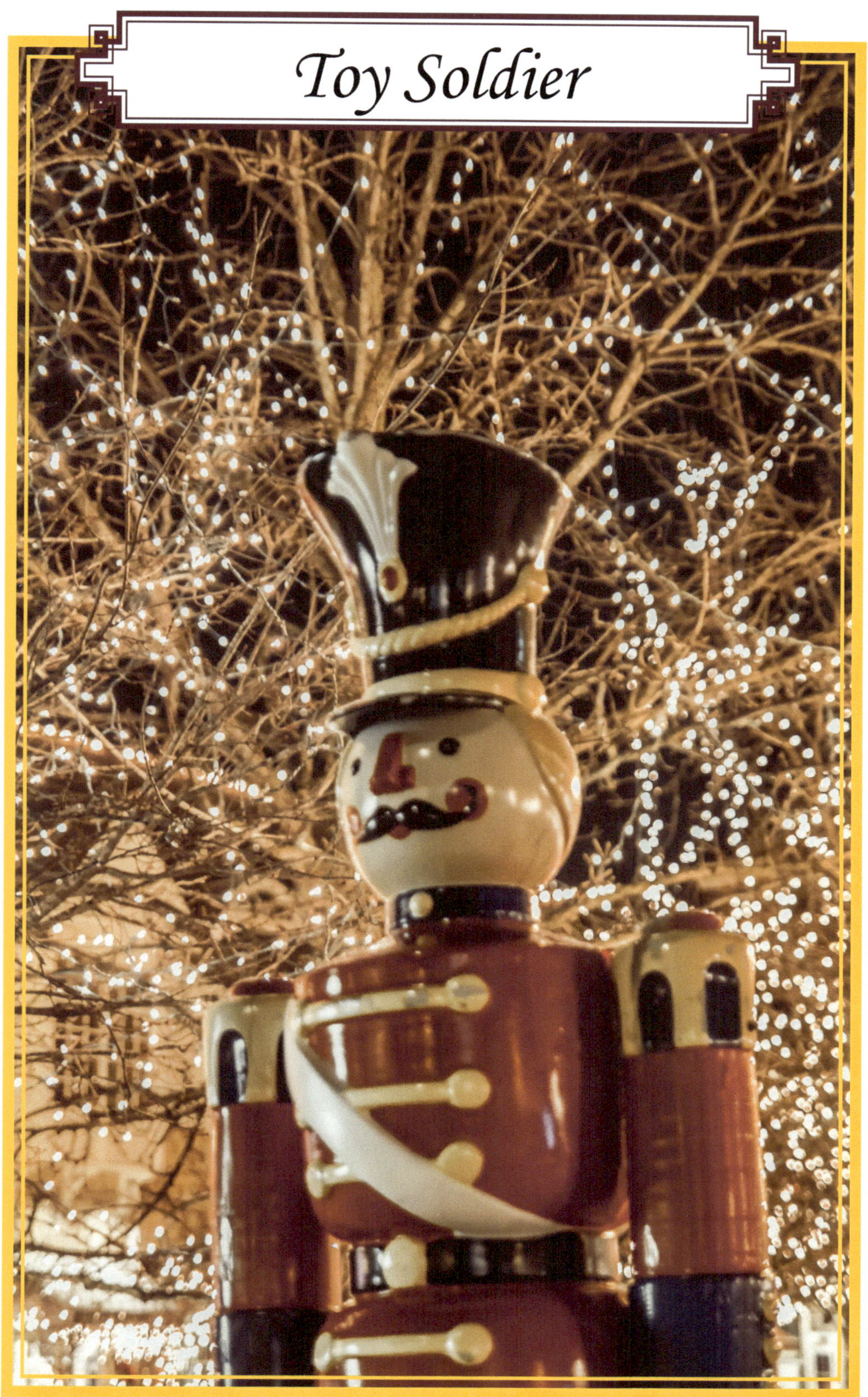

Decorating the Tree

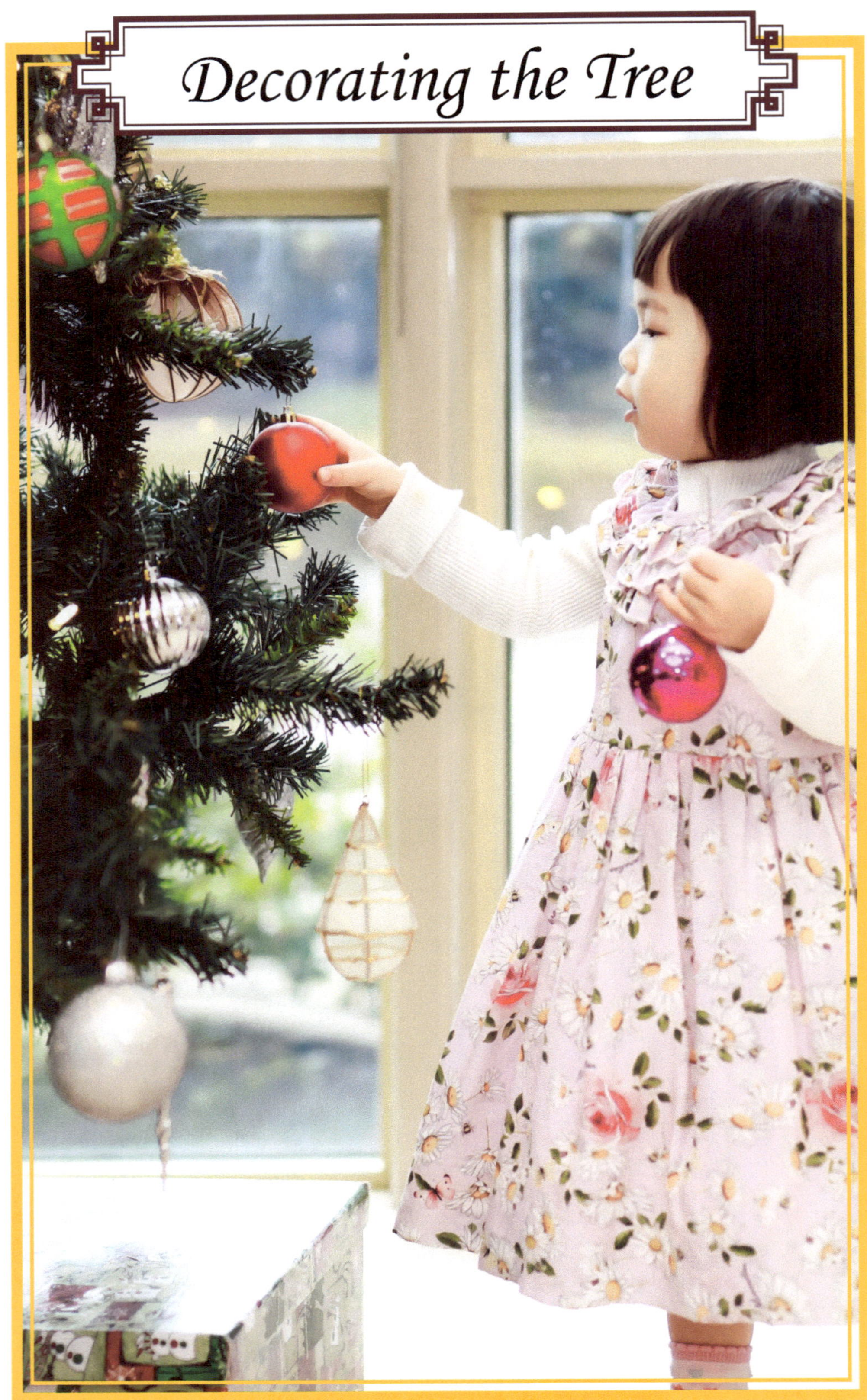

Merry and Bright

The First Noel

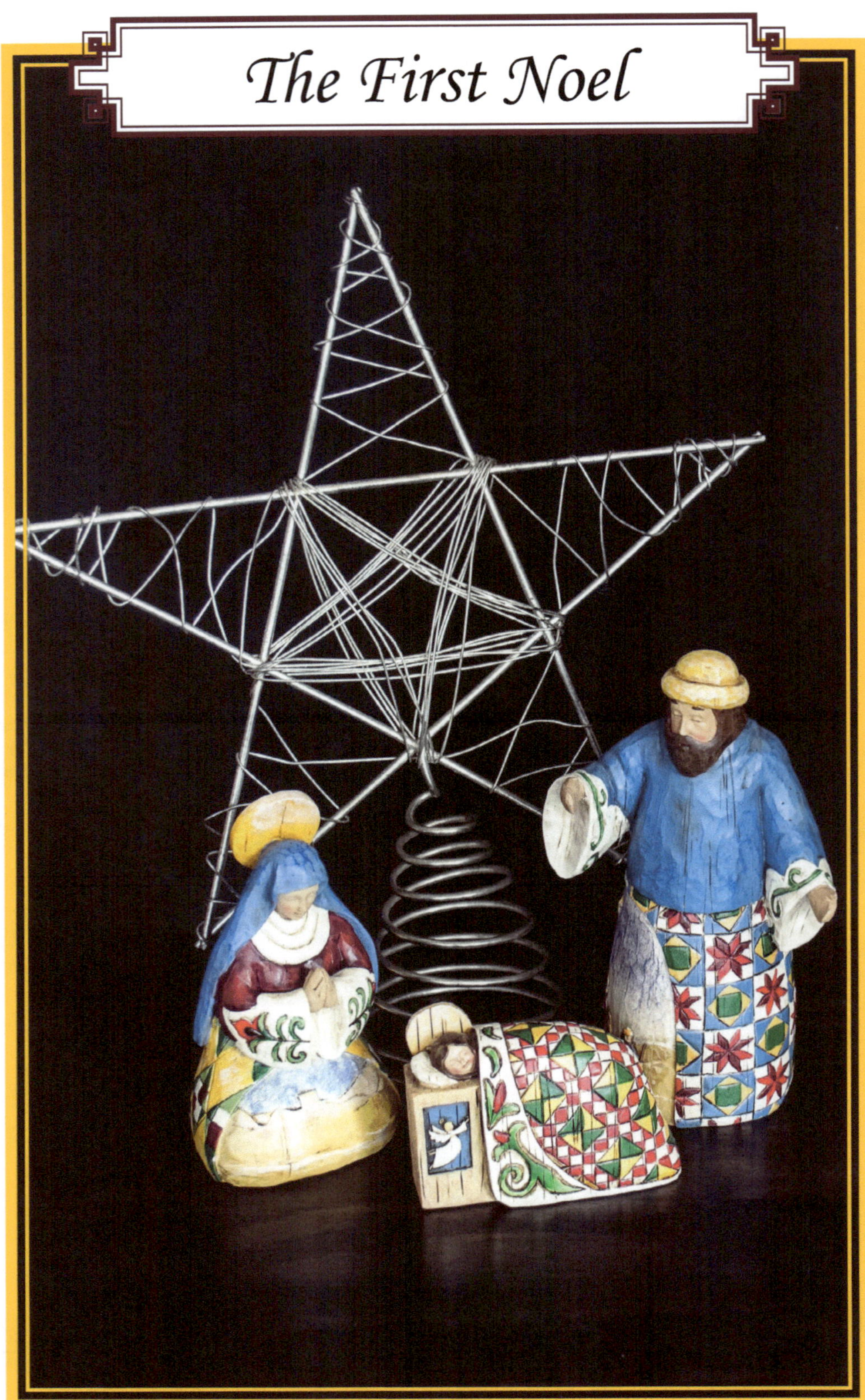

Christmas Greetings

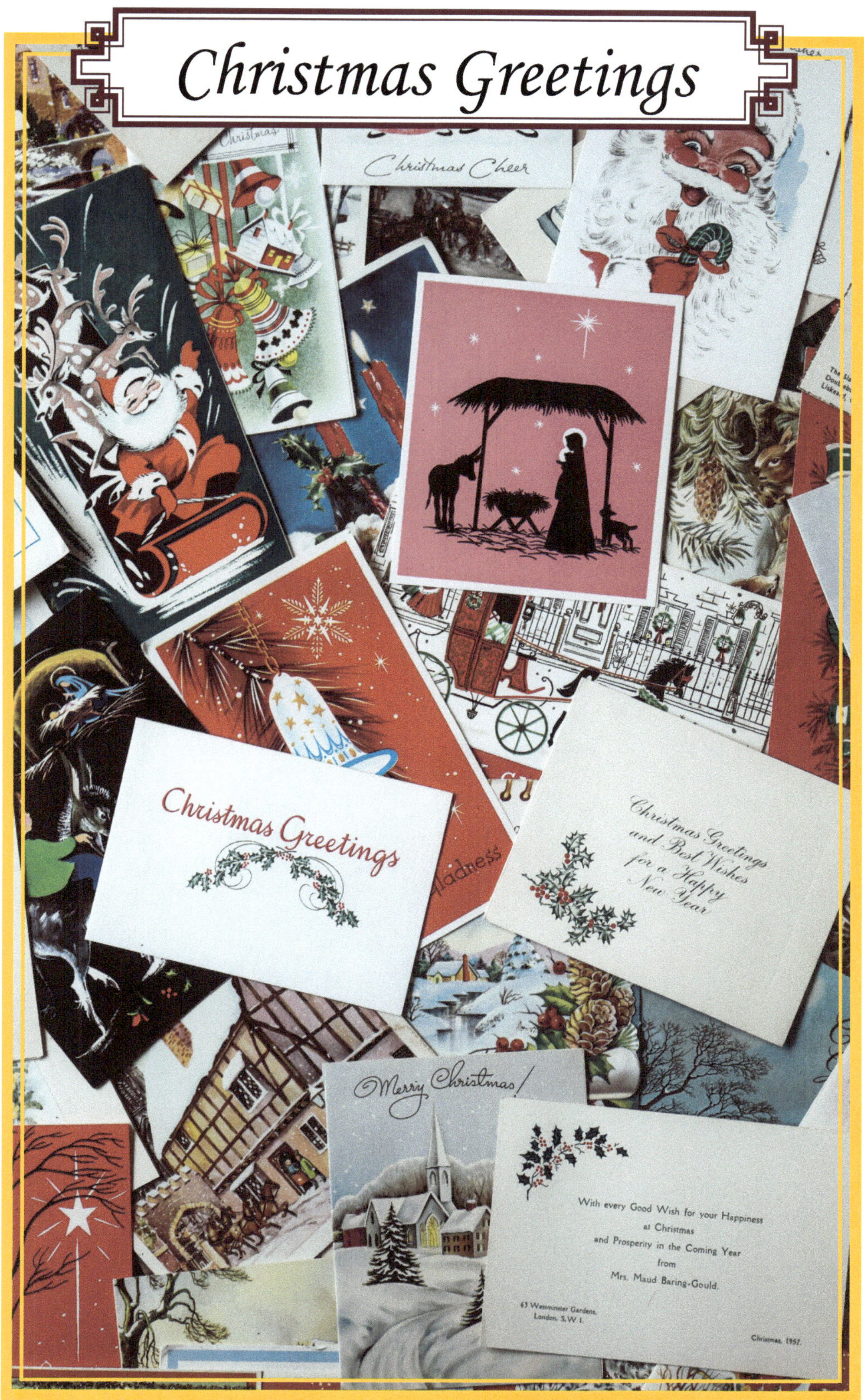

Beautiful Poinsettias

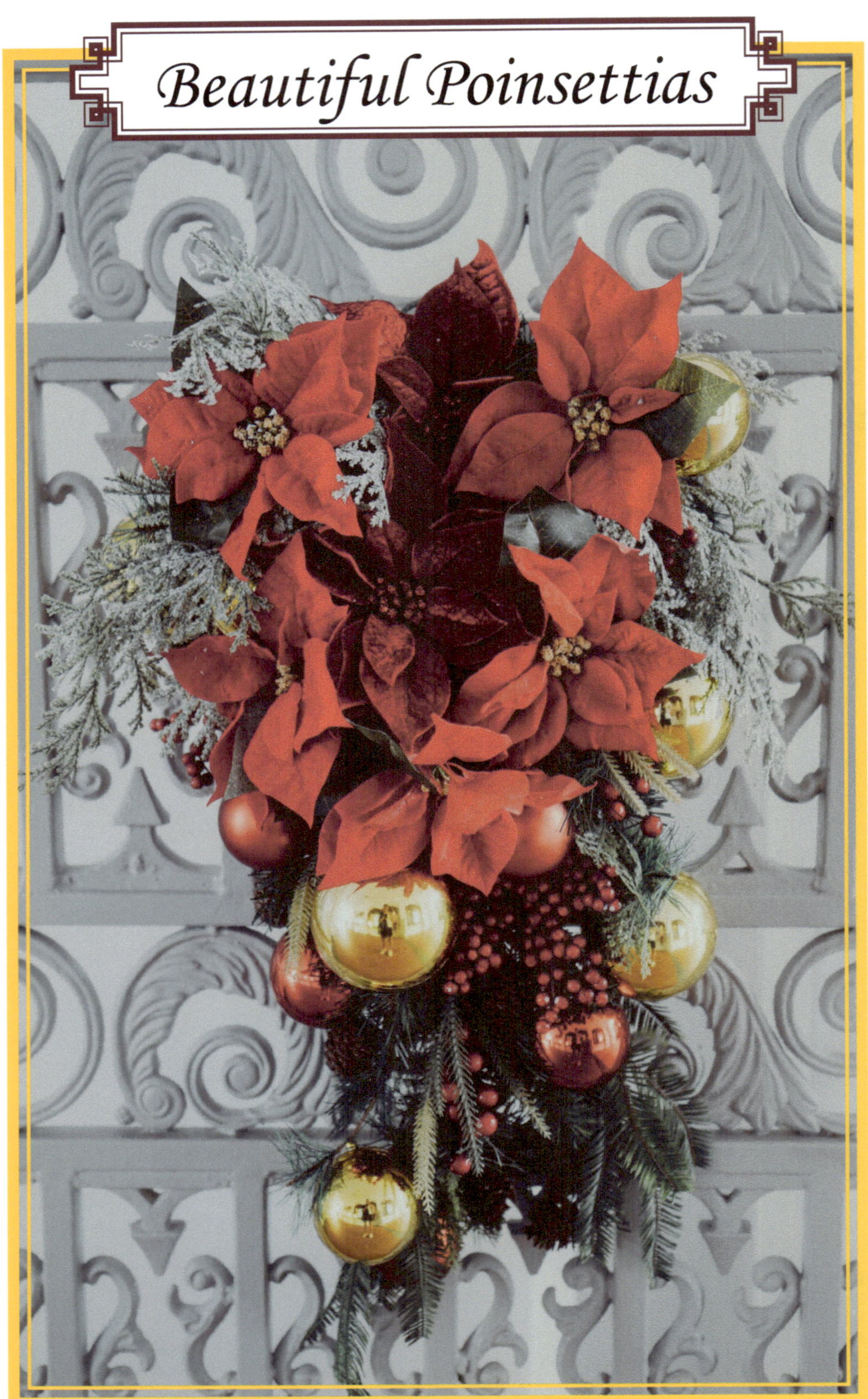

Candy Canes

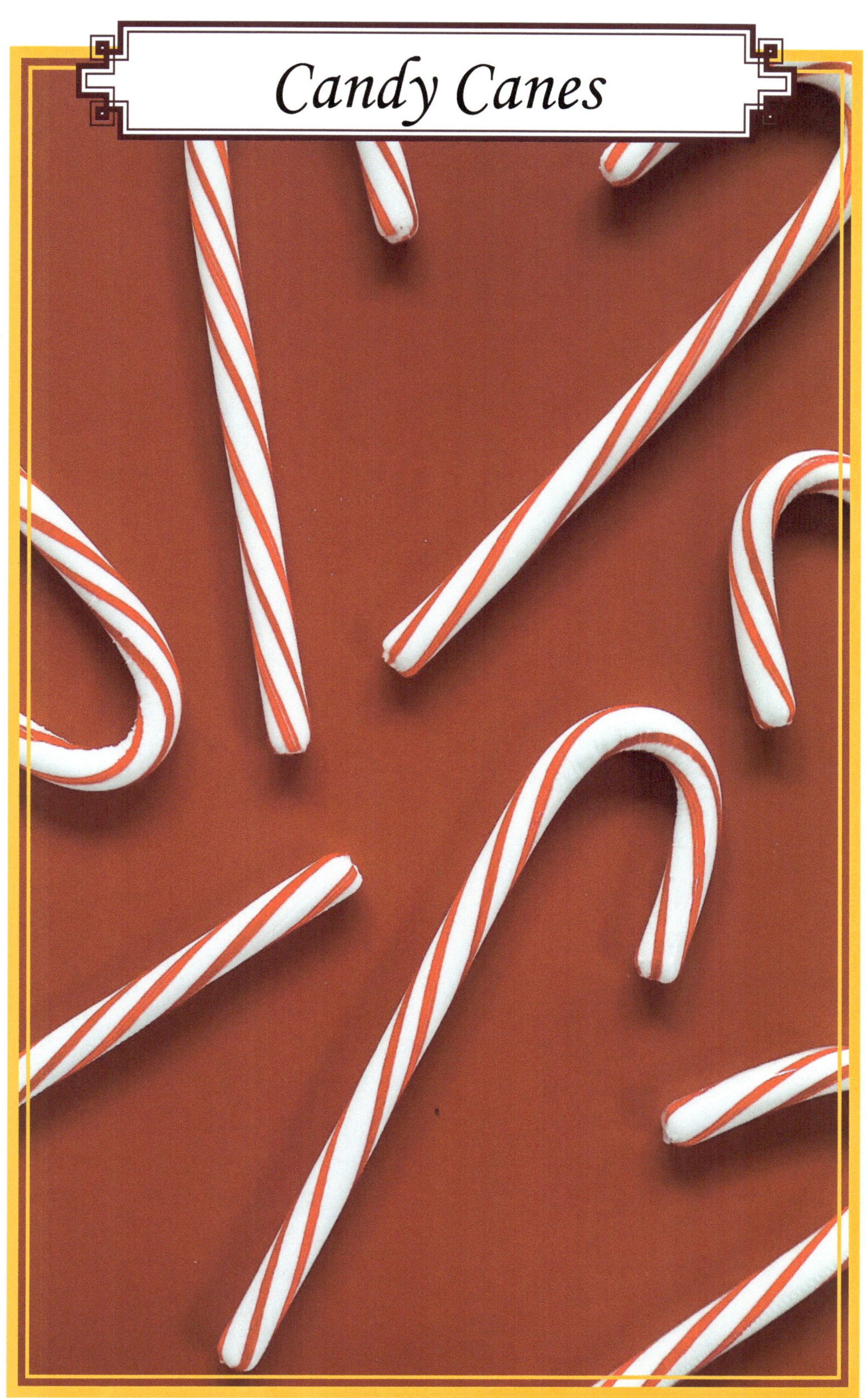

Checking It Twice

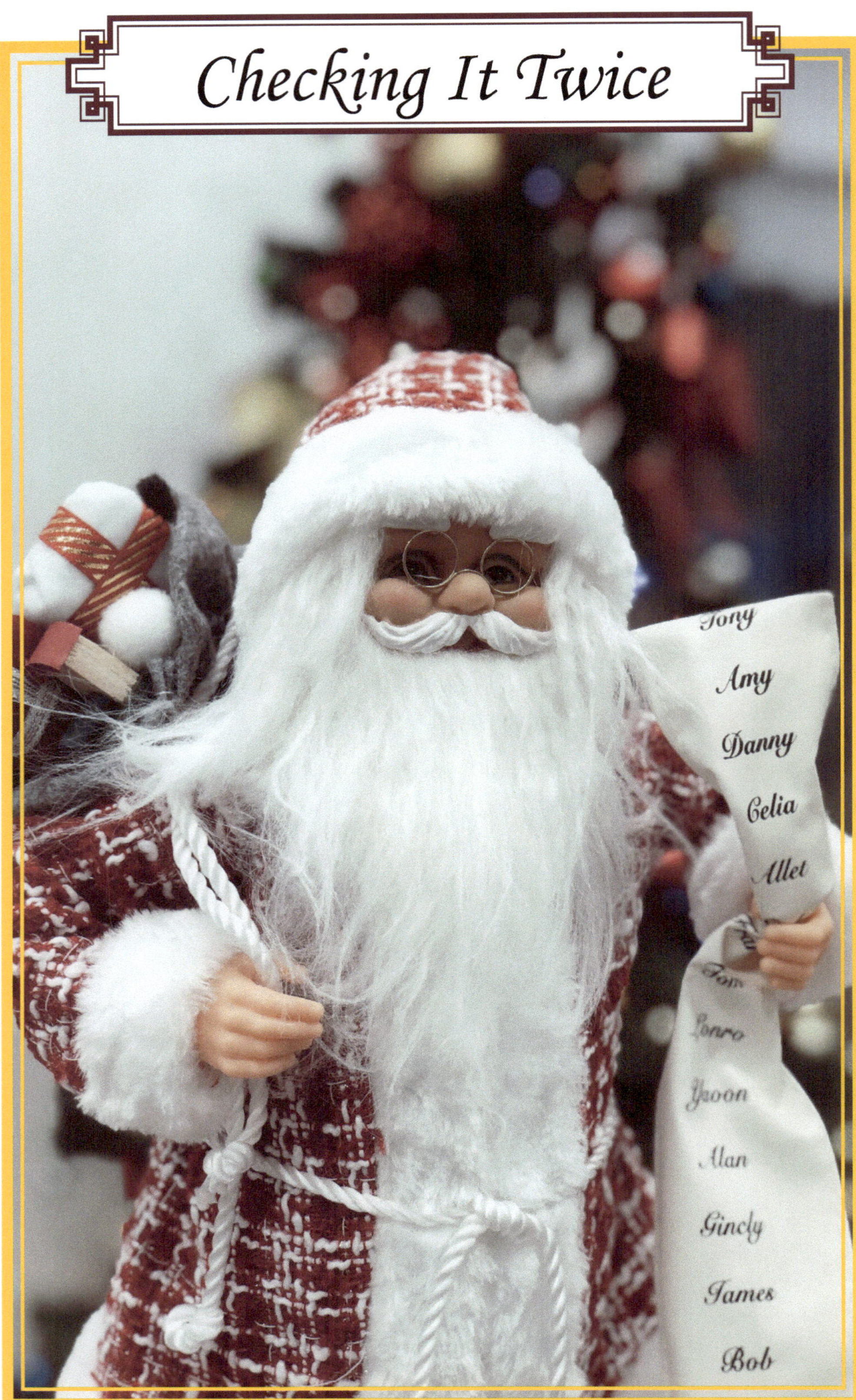

Cookies for Santa

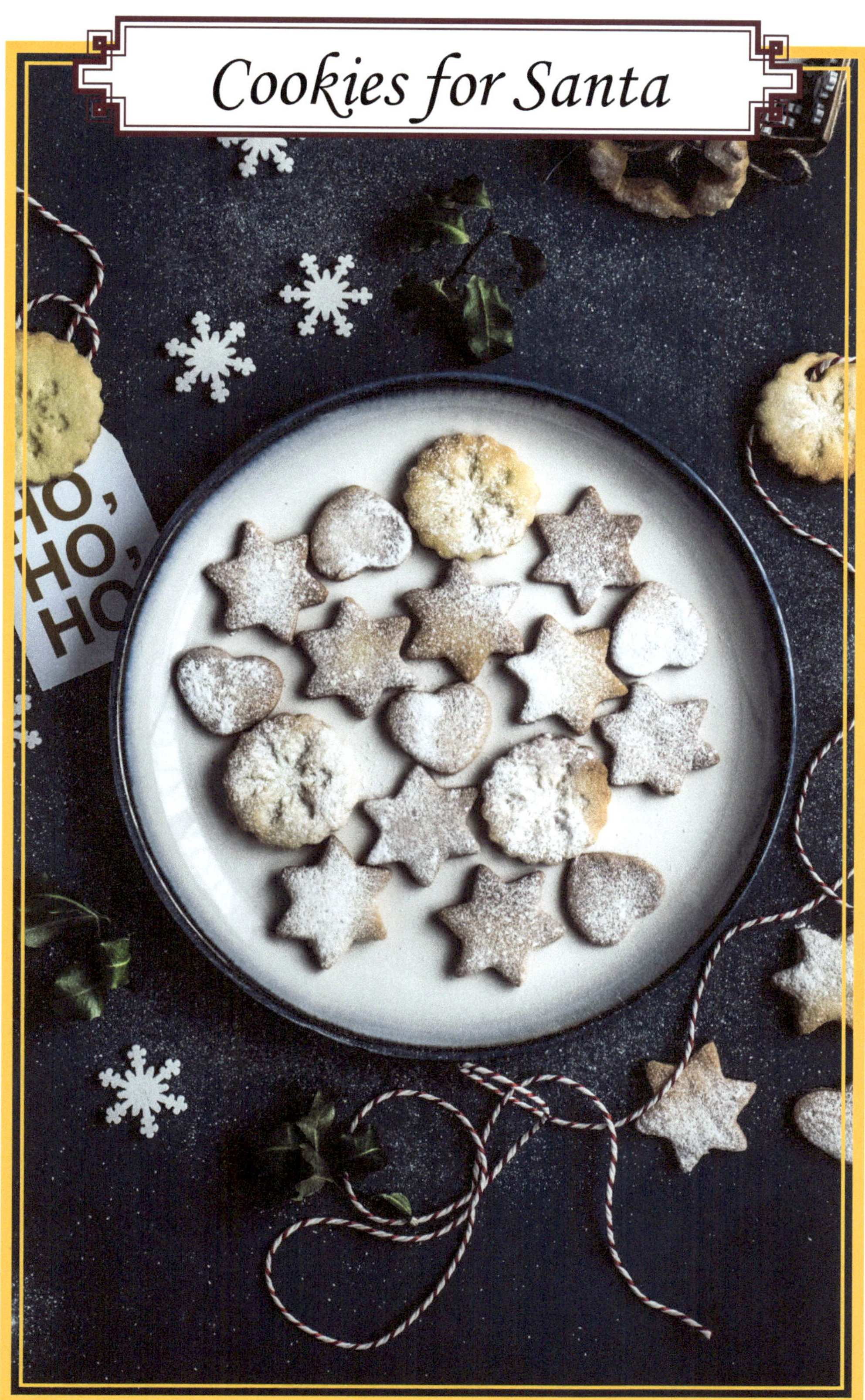

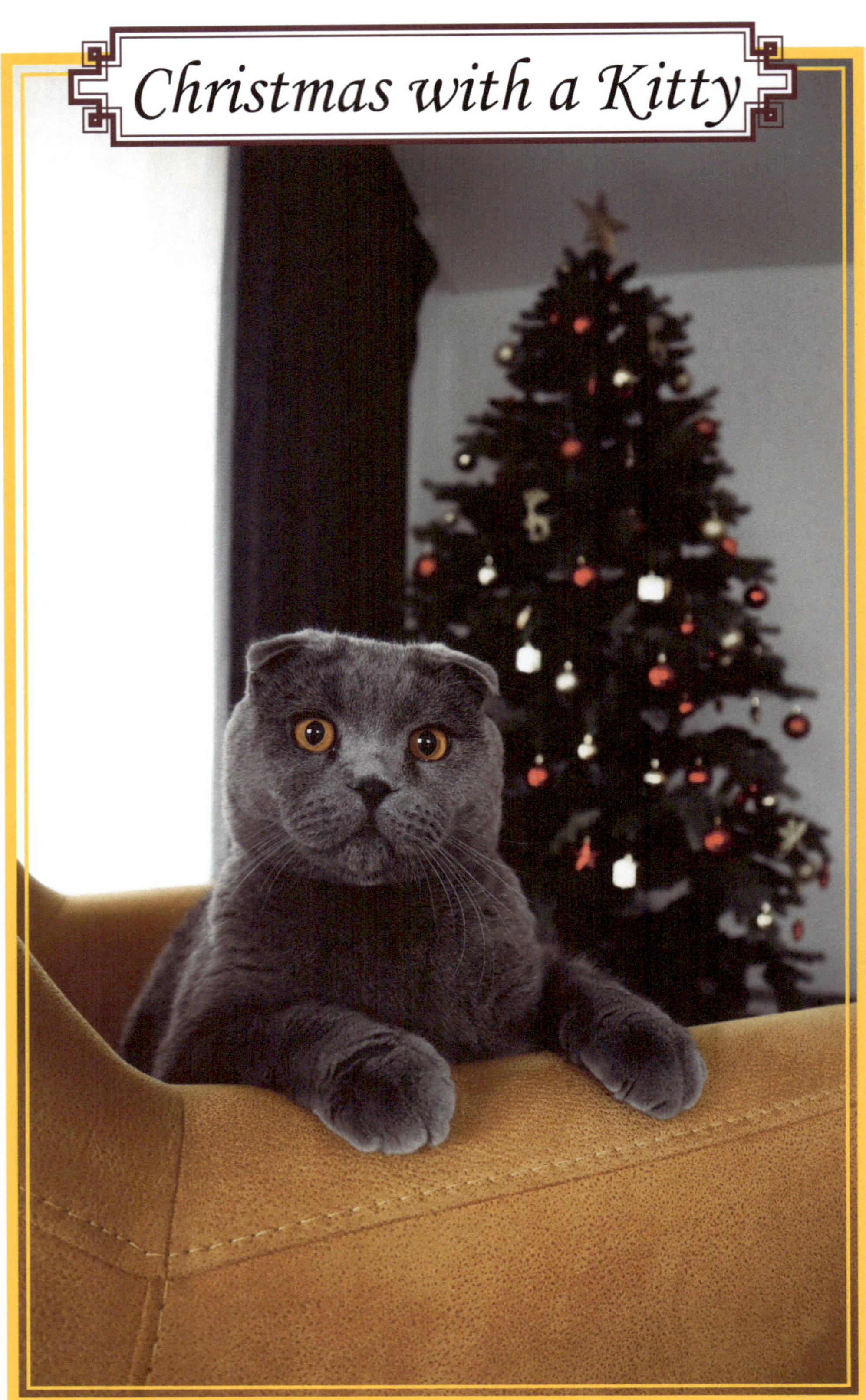
Christmas with a Kitty

Christmas Traditions

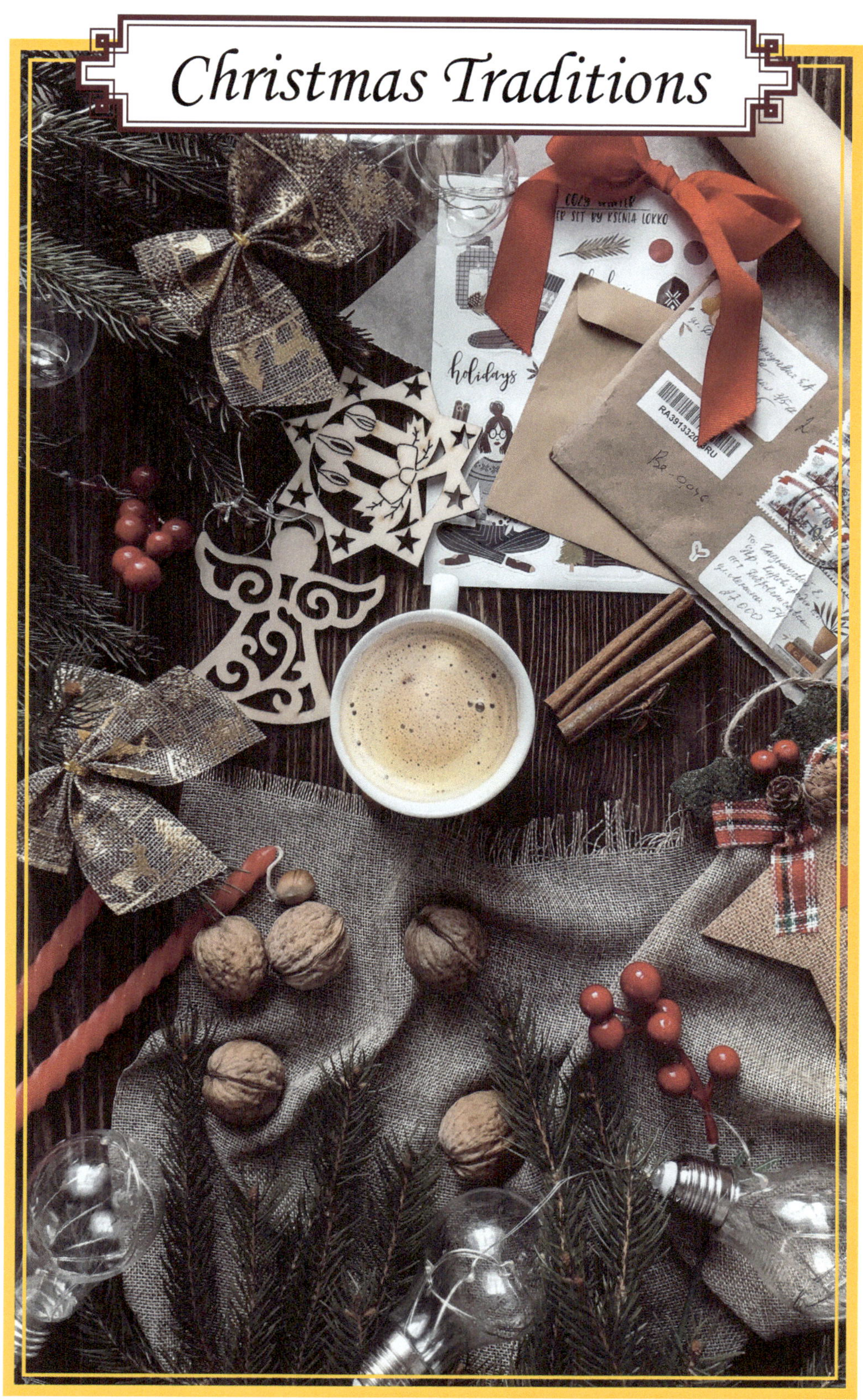

Cute Sweater

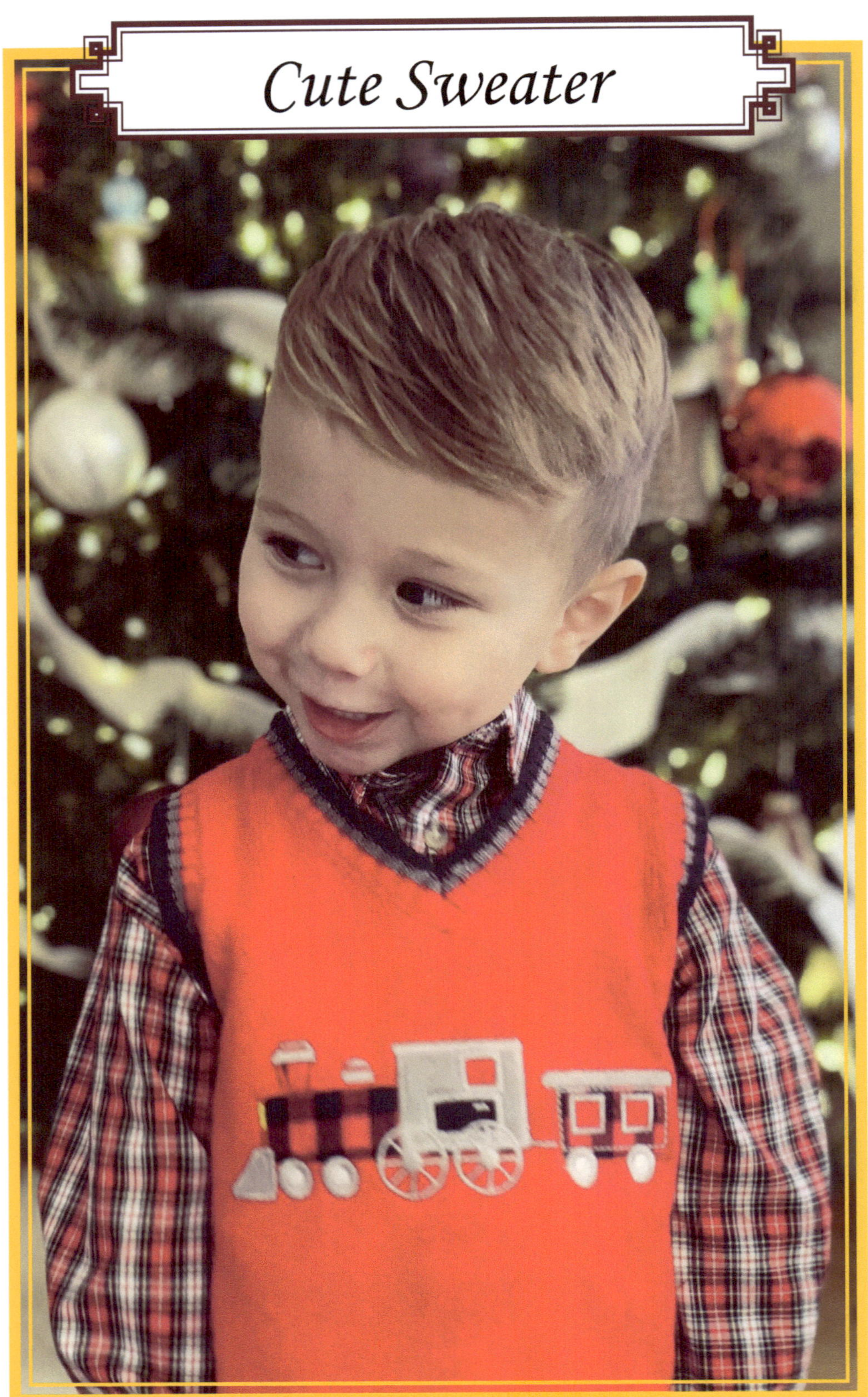

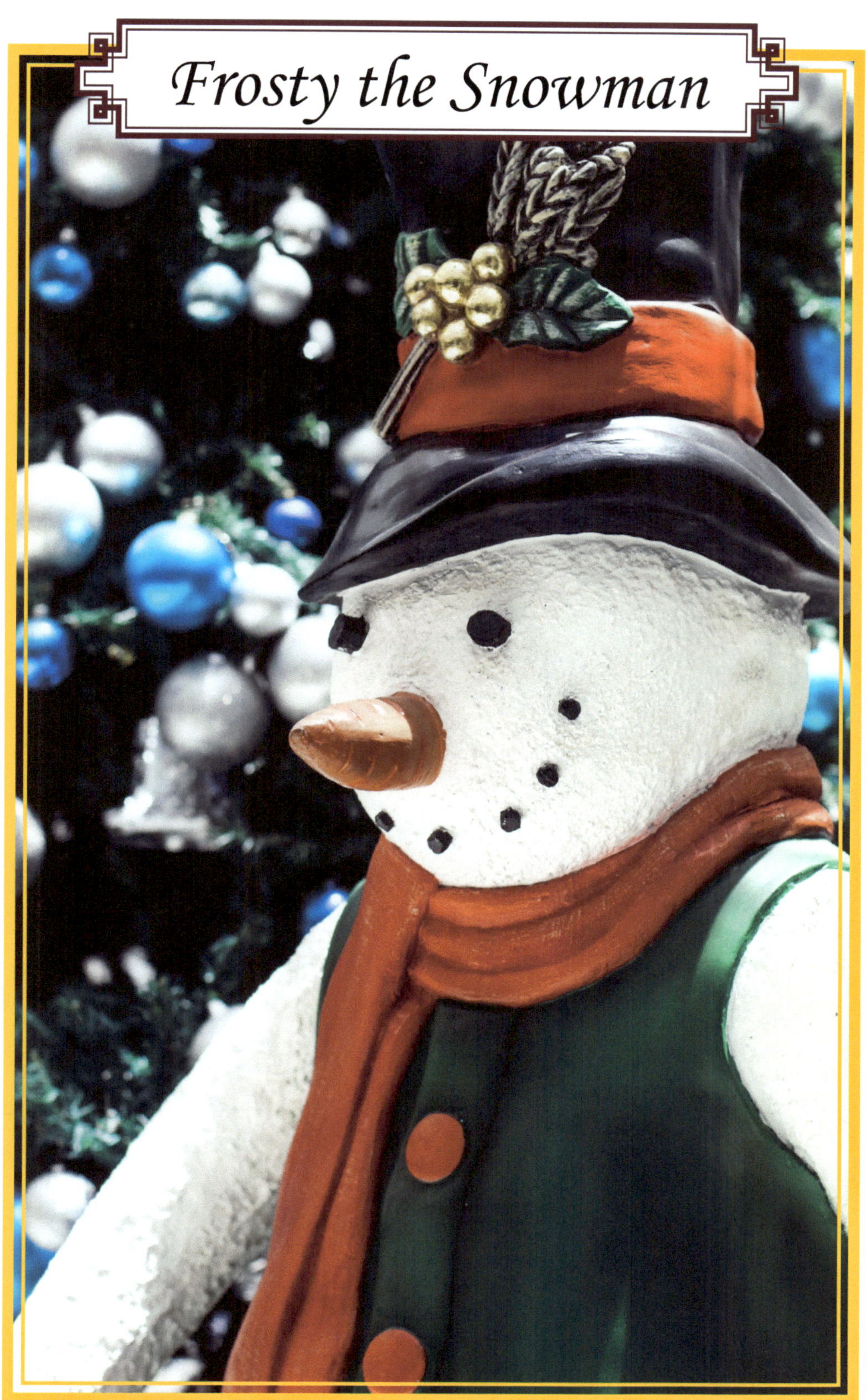

Frosty the Snowman

Is It a Dog or an Elf?

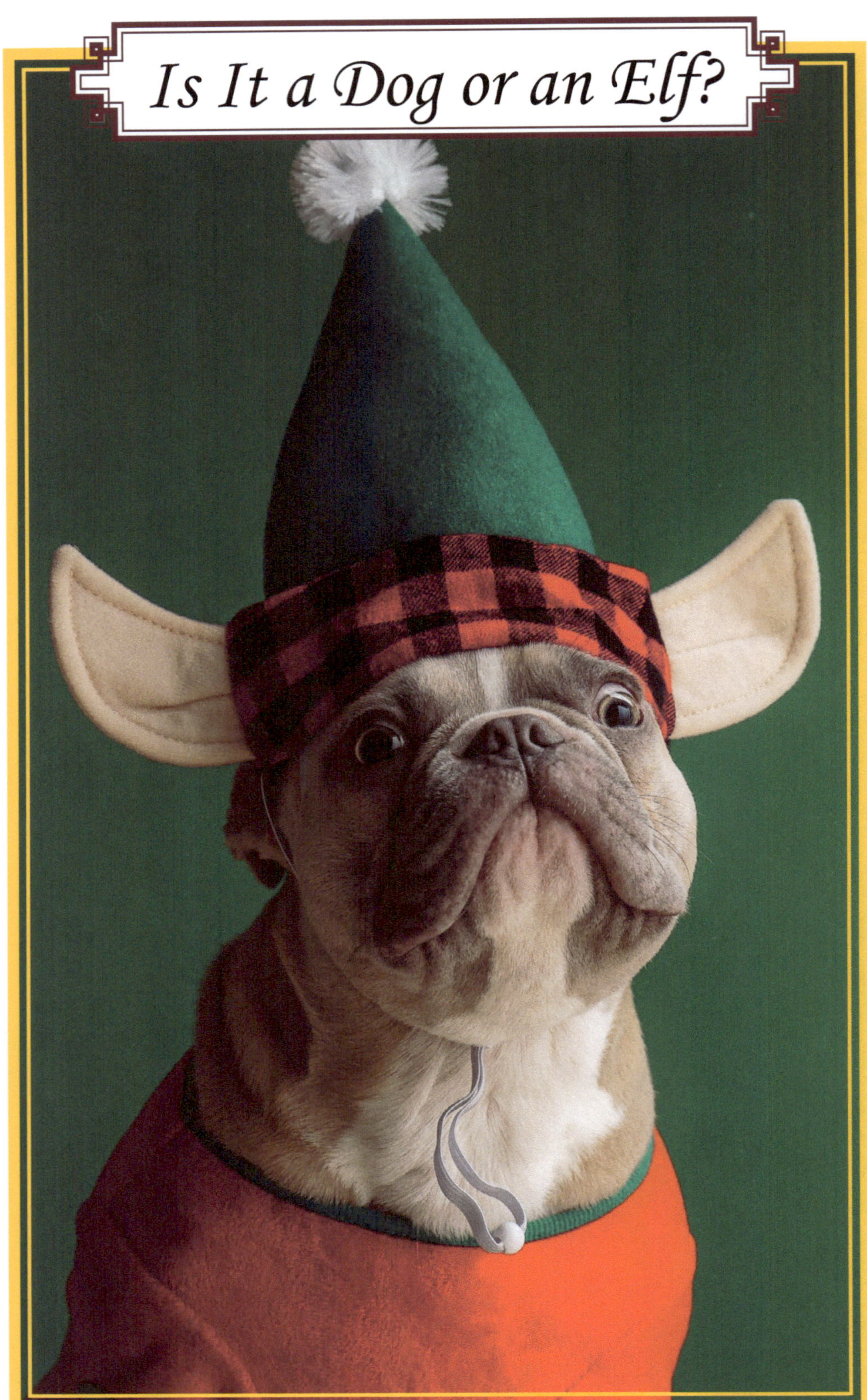

Rudolph

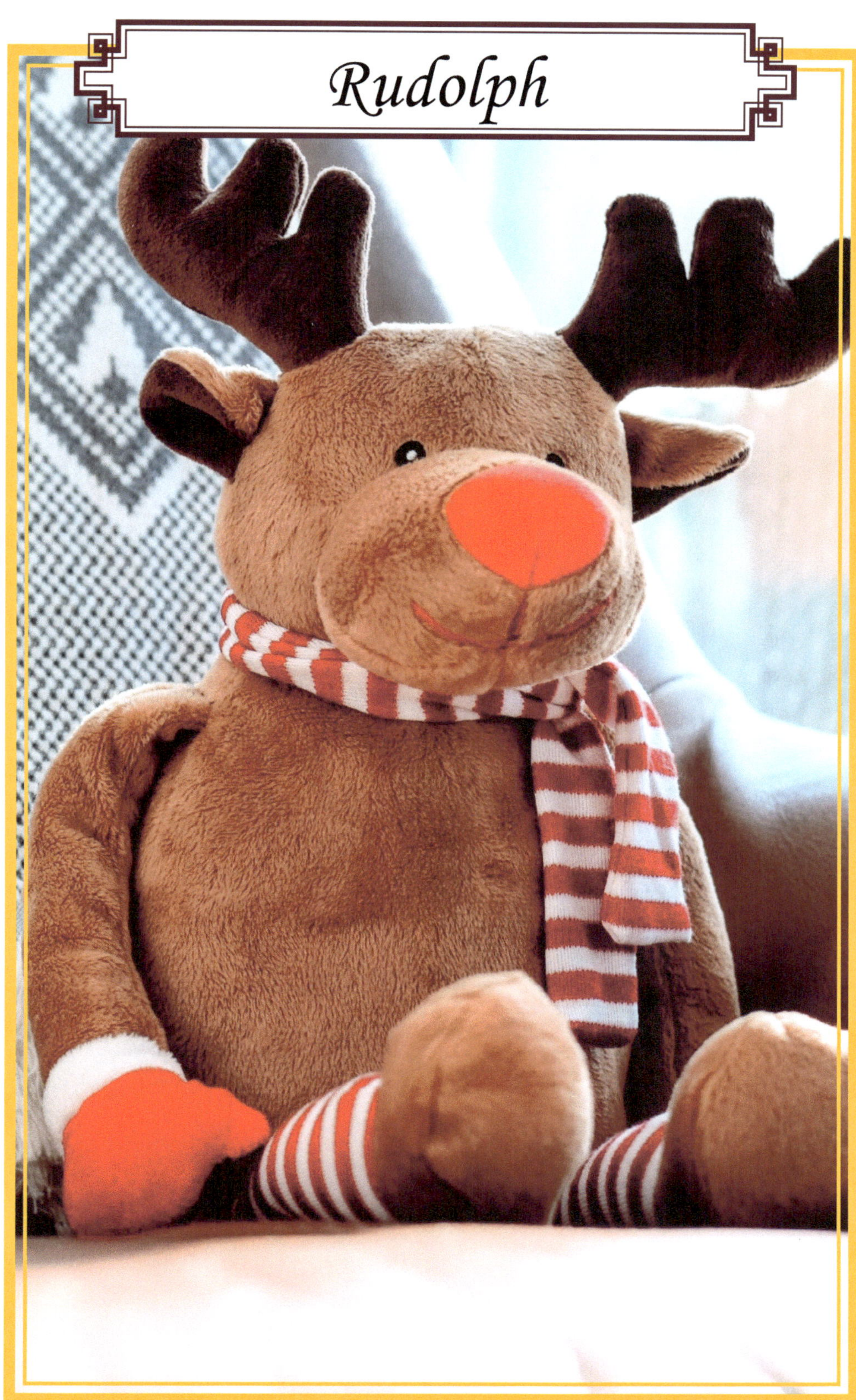

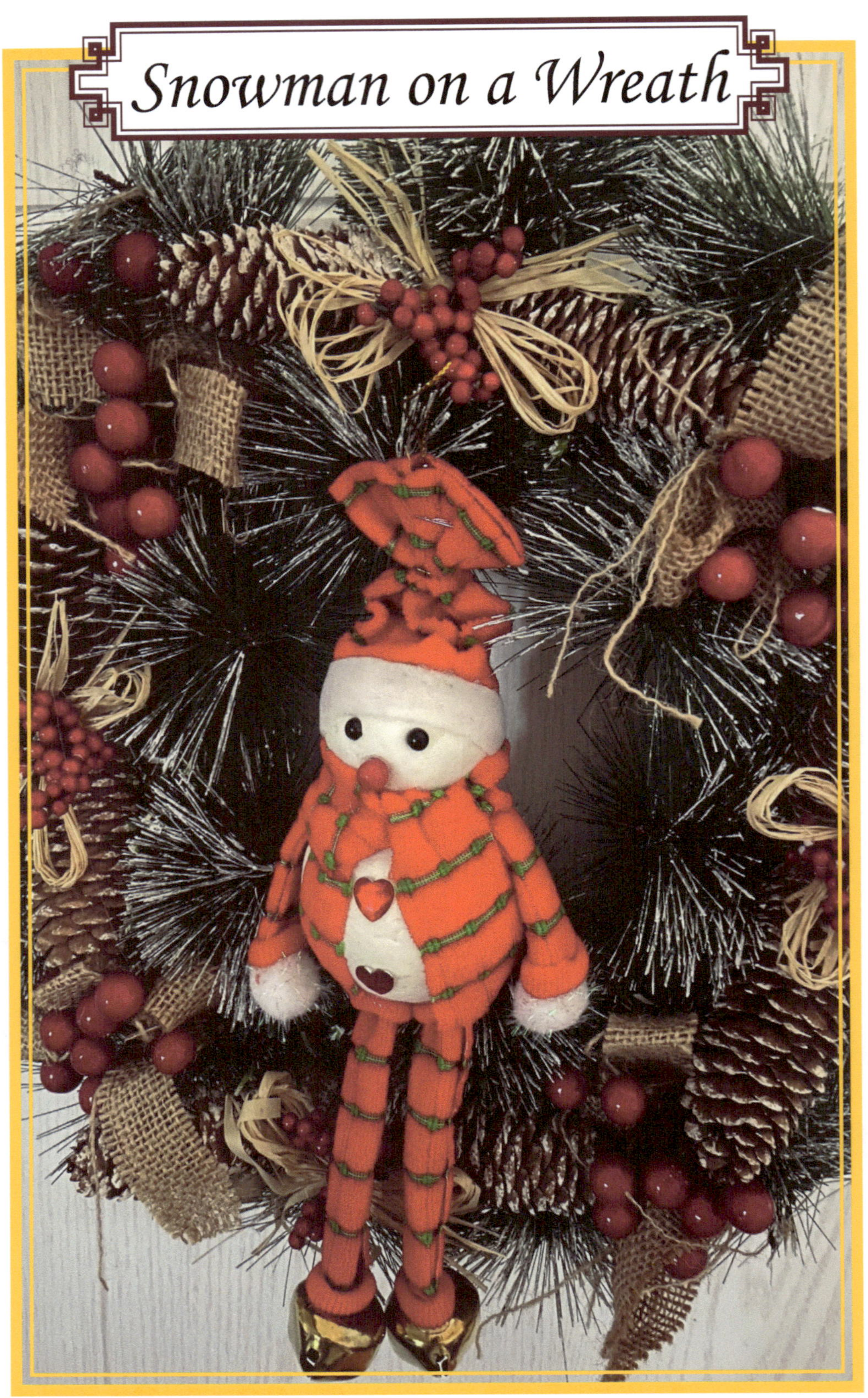

Snowman on a Wreath

Outdoor Decorations

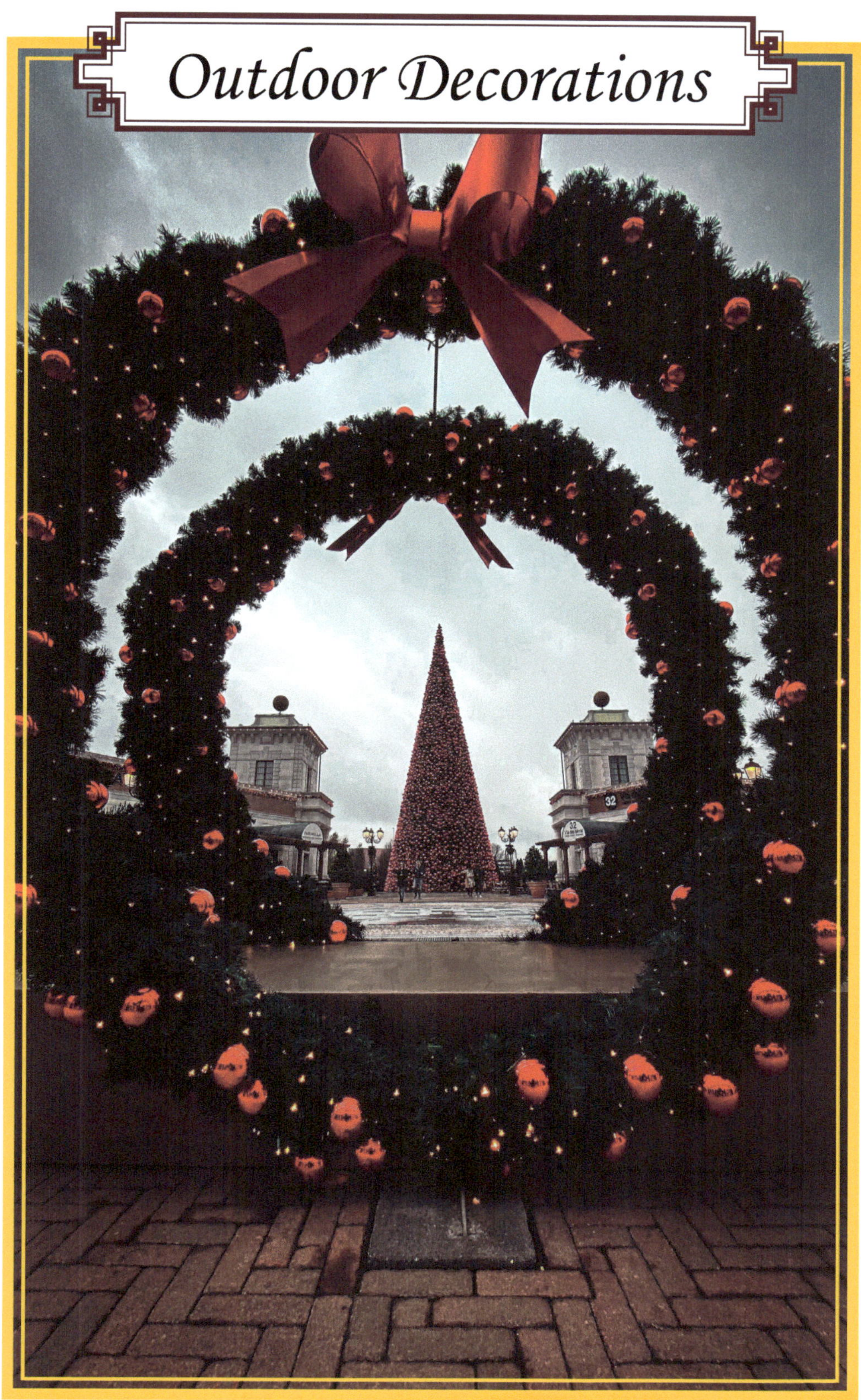

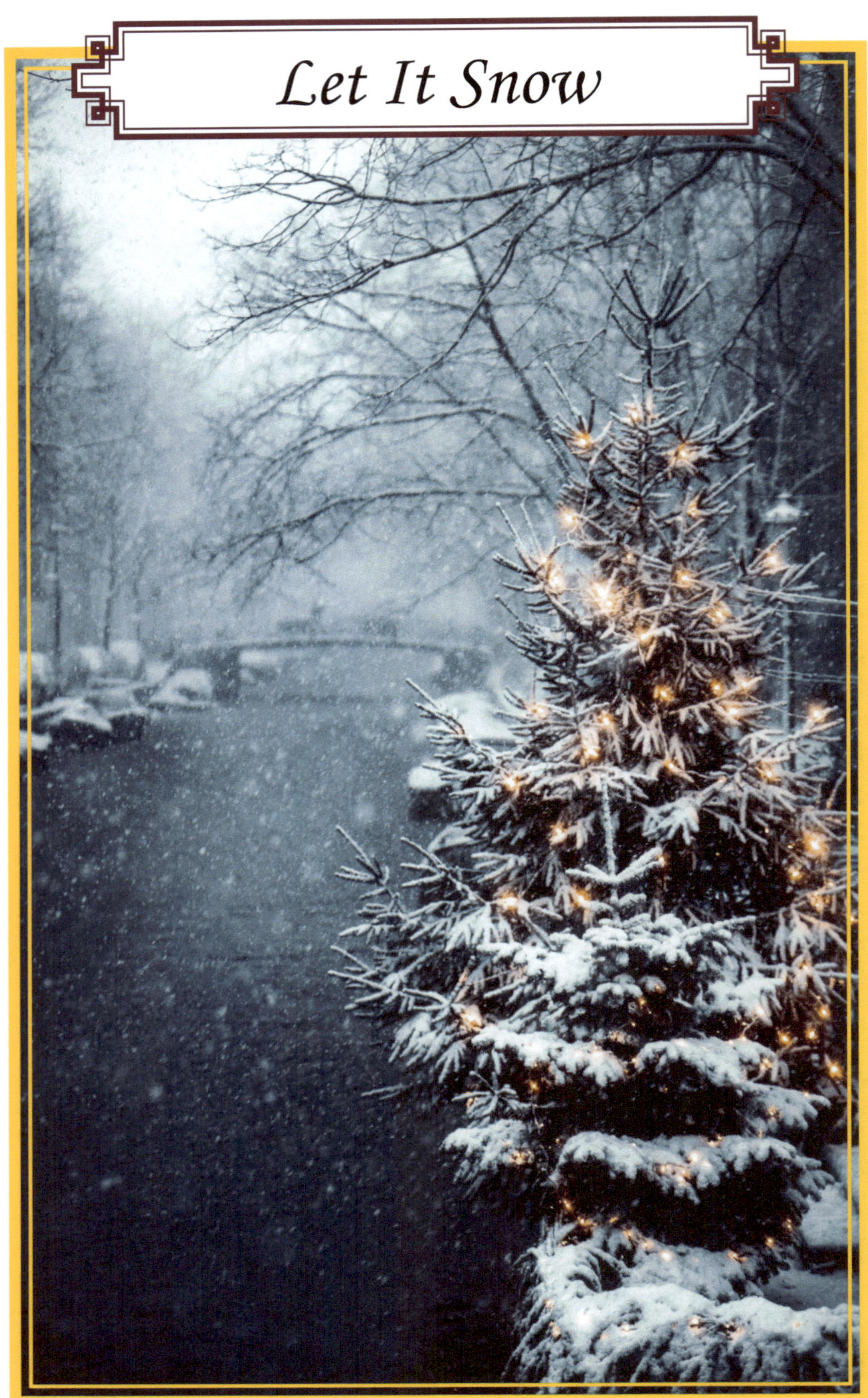
Let It Snow

O Holy Night

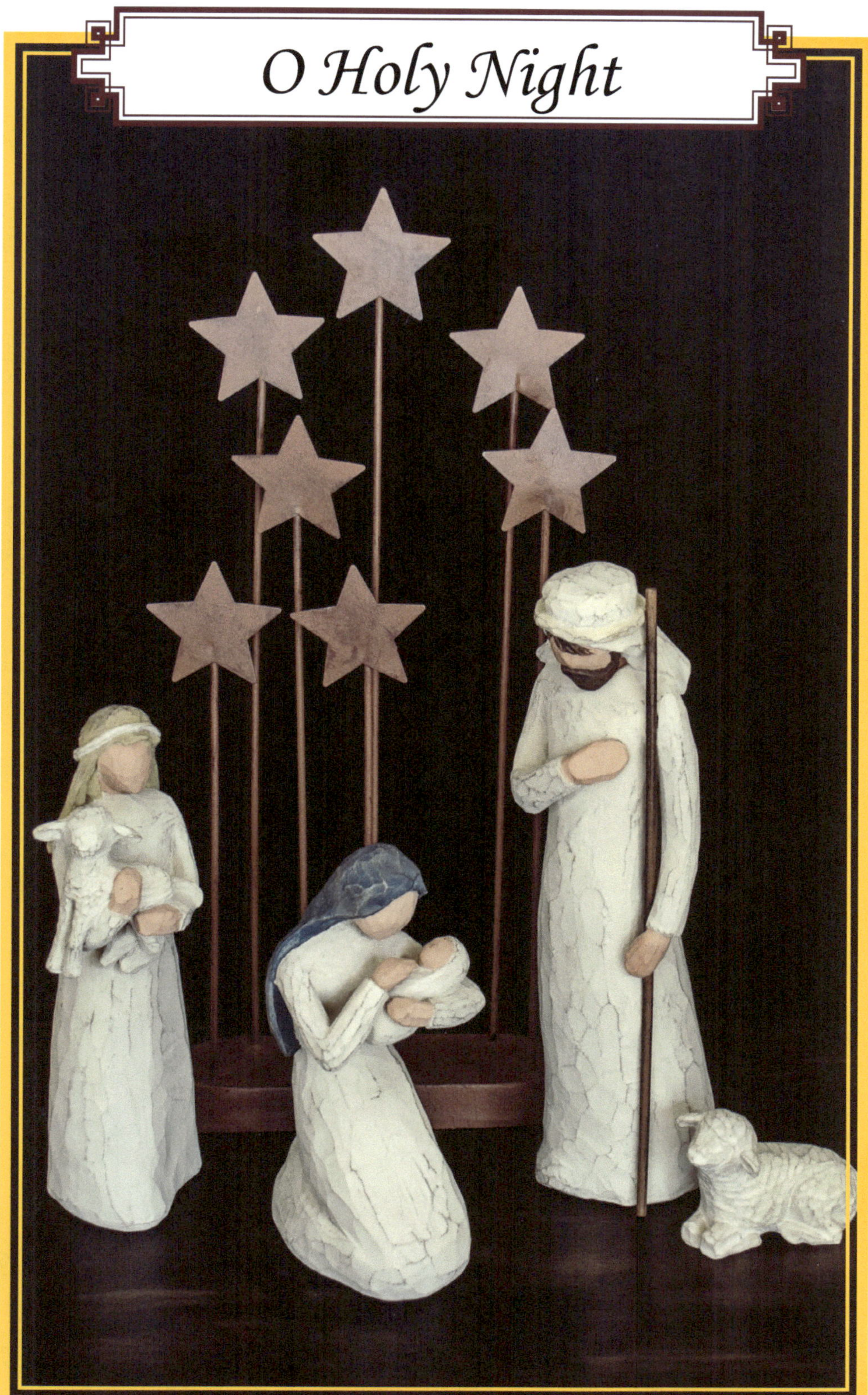

Gifts Under the Tree

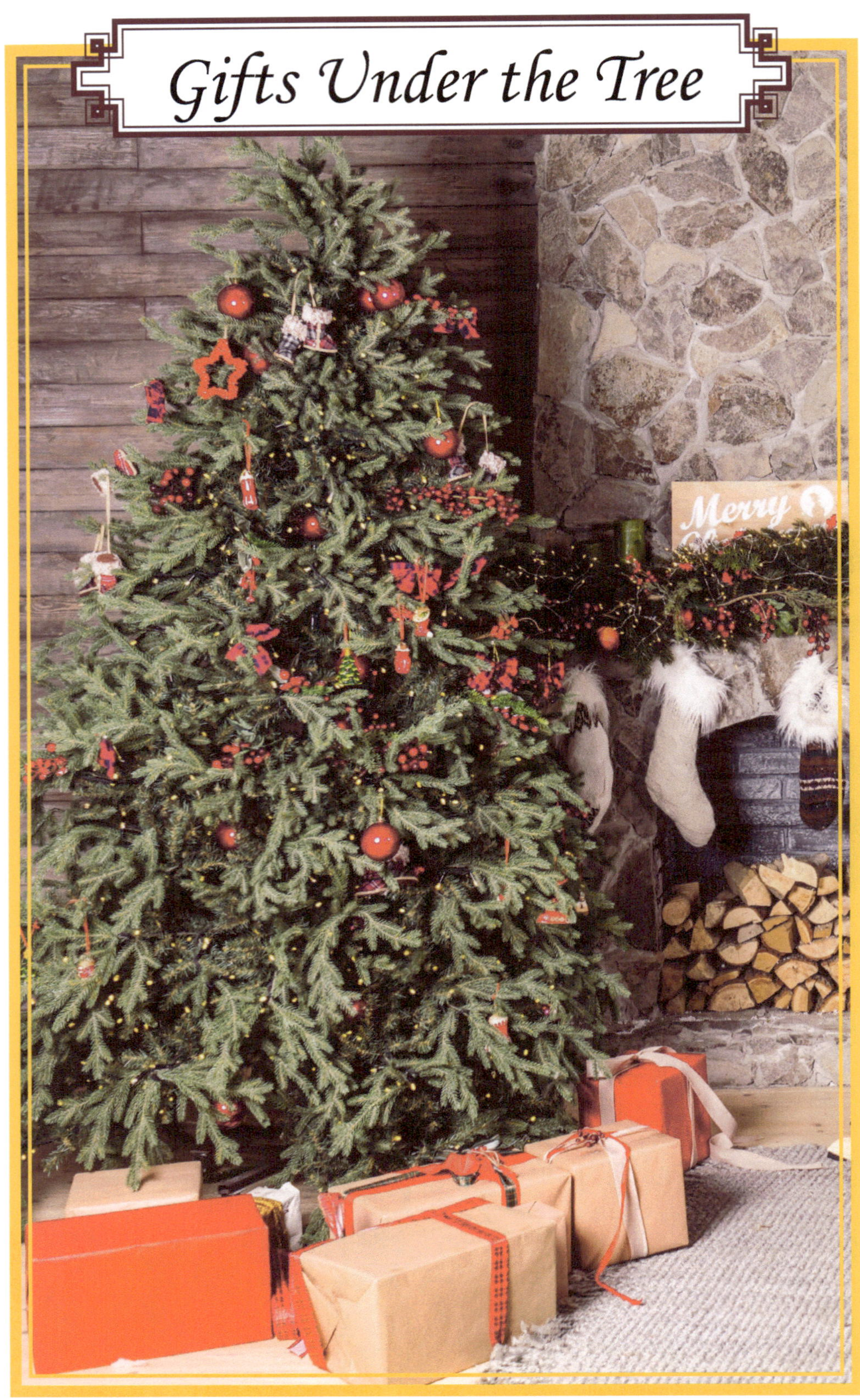

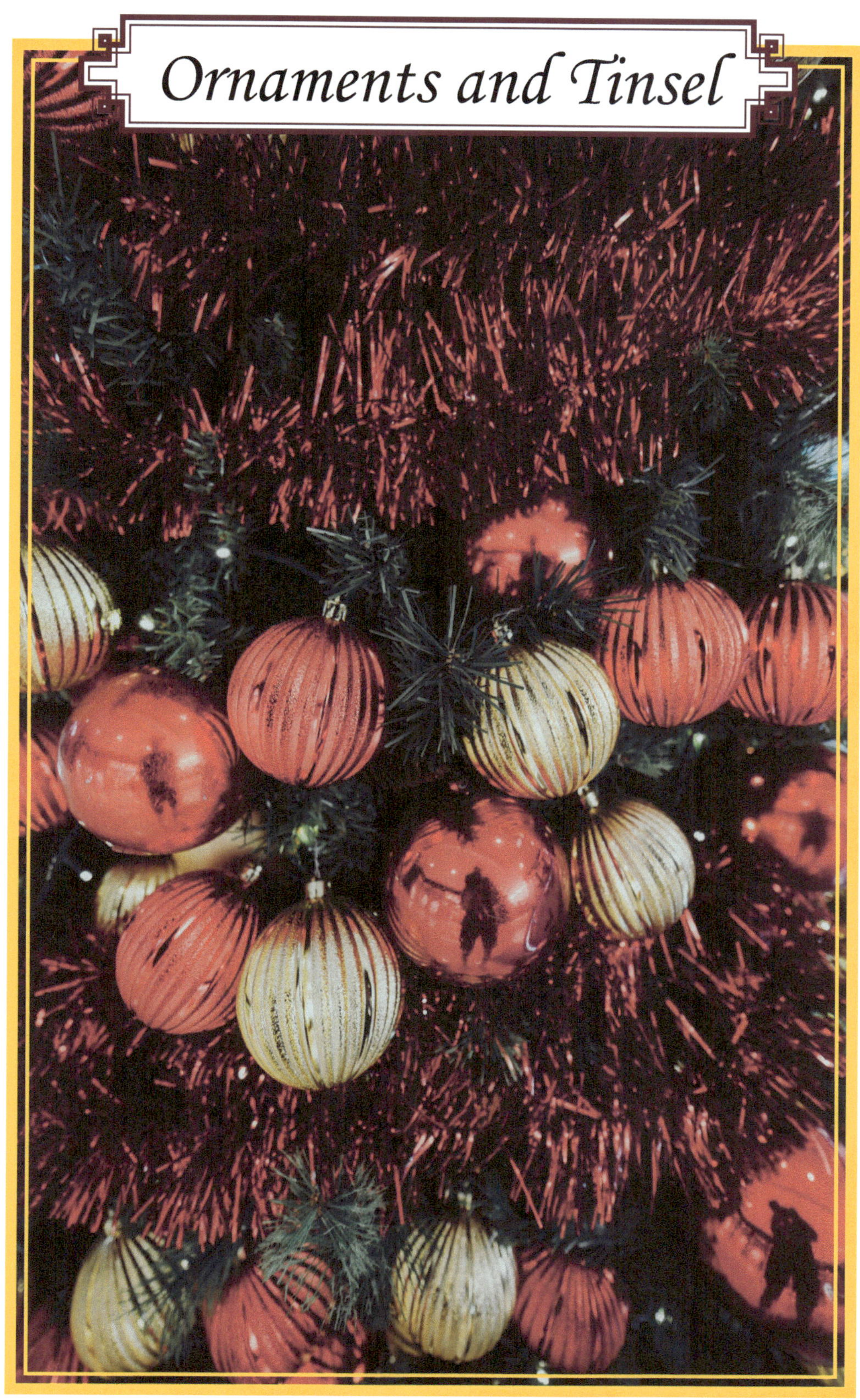
Ornaments and Tinsel

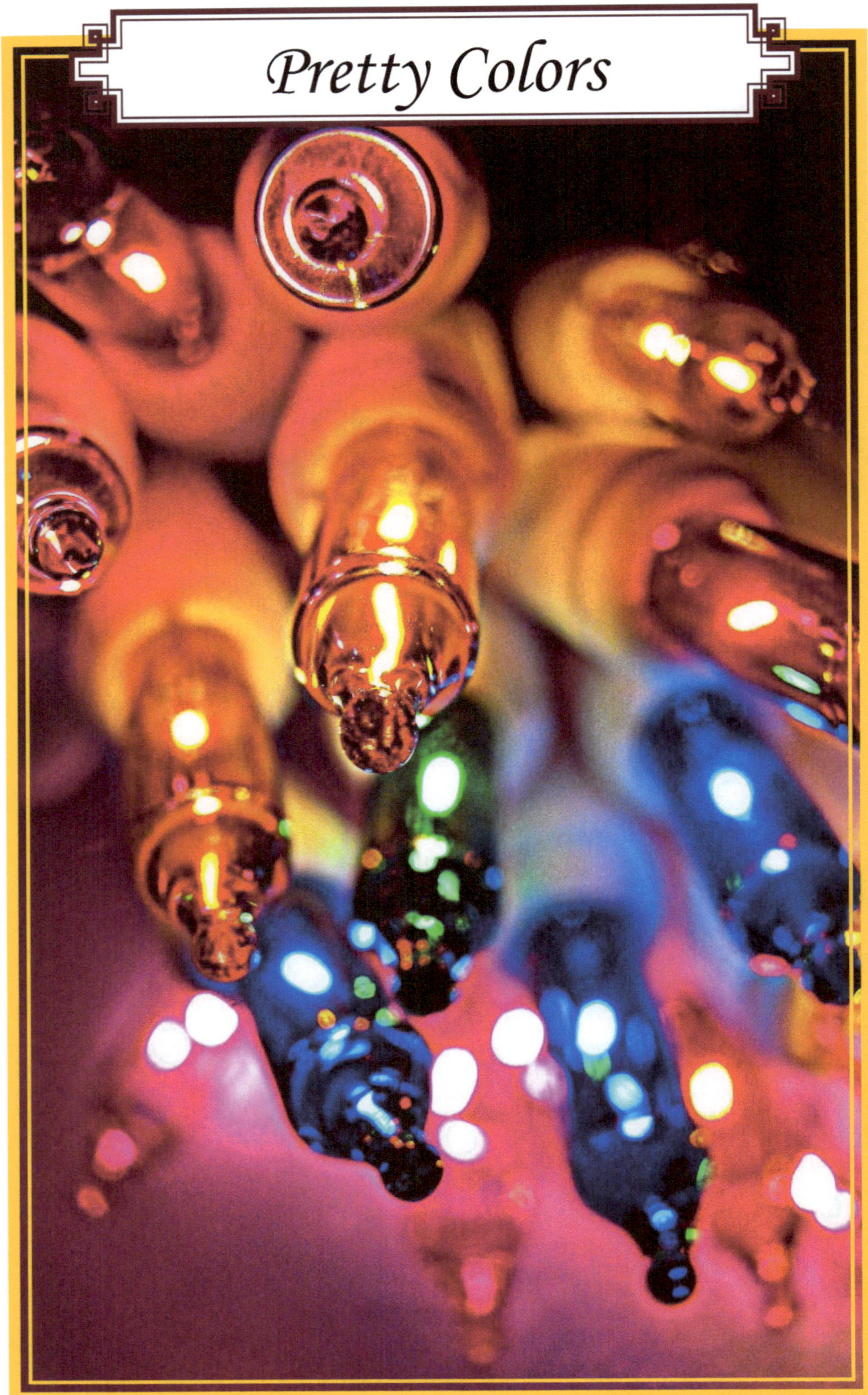
Pretty Colors

The Nutcracker

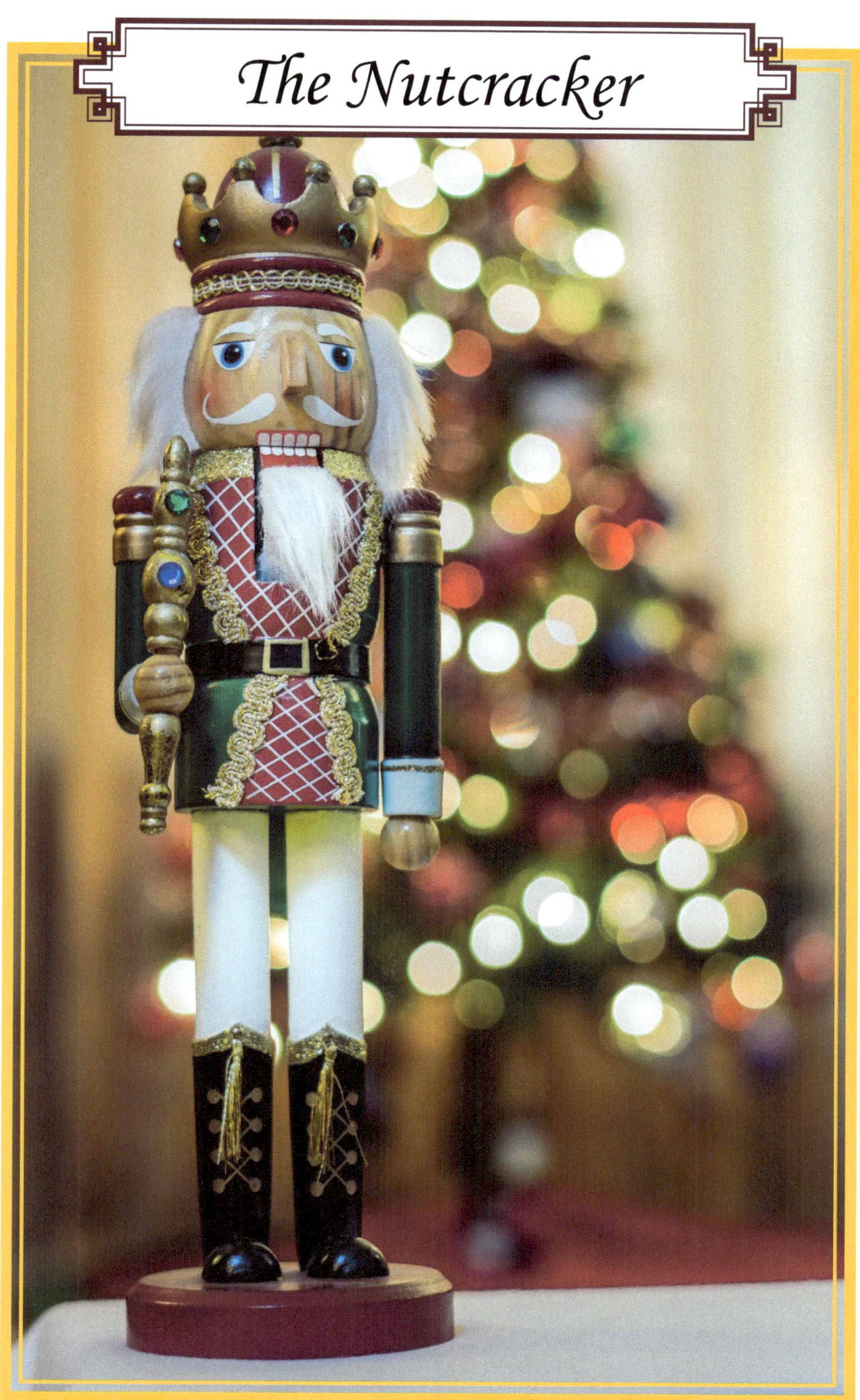

Joy of the Season

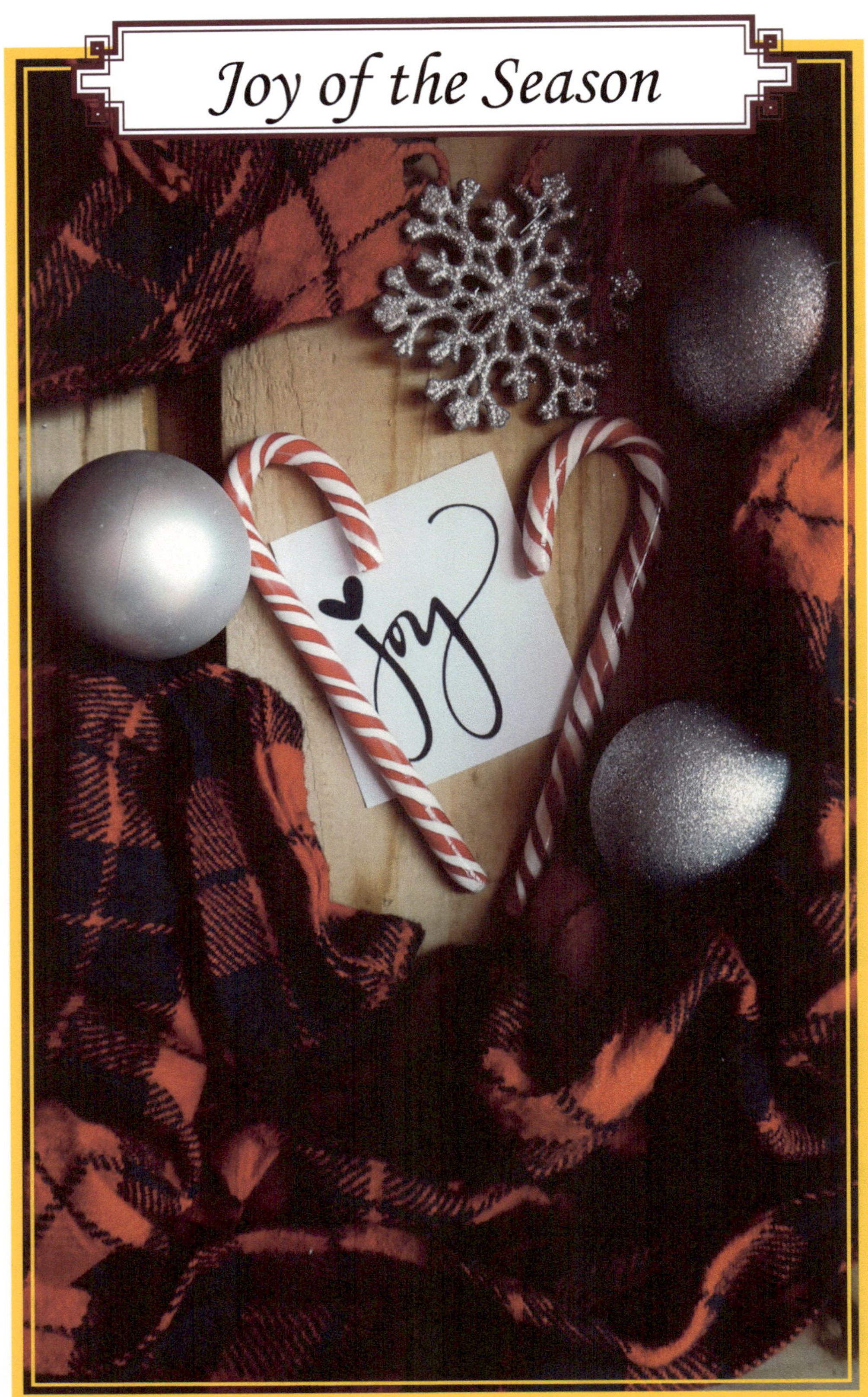

The Star on the Tree

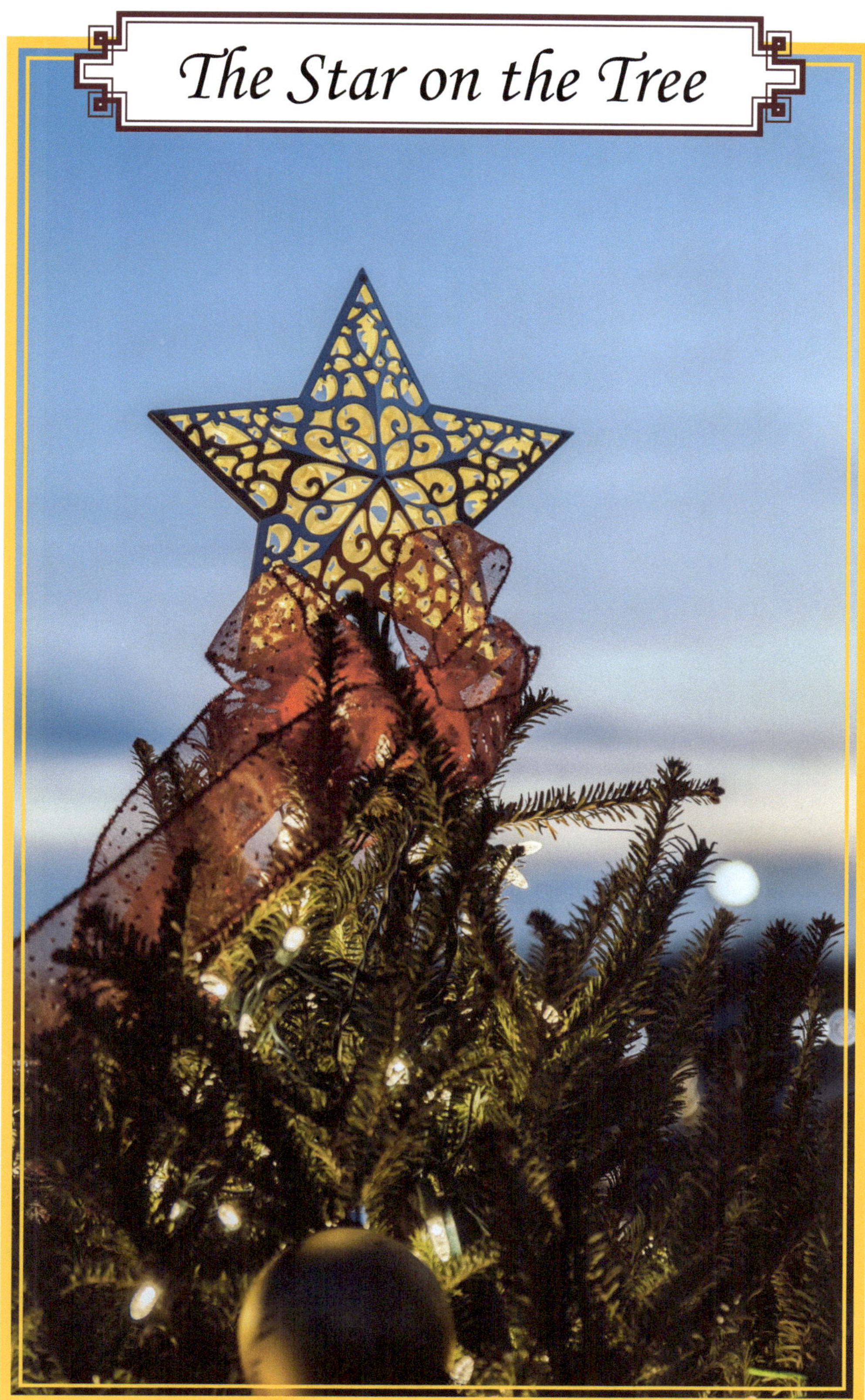

Warm Chestnuts

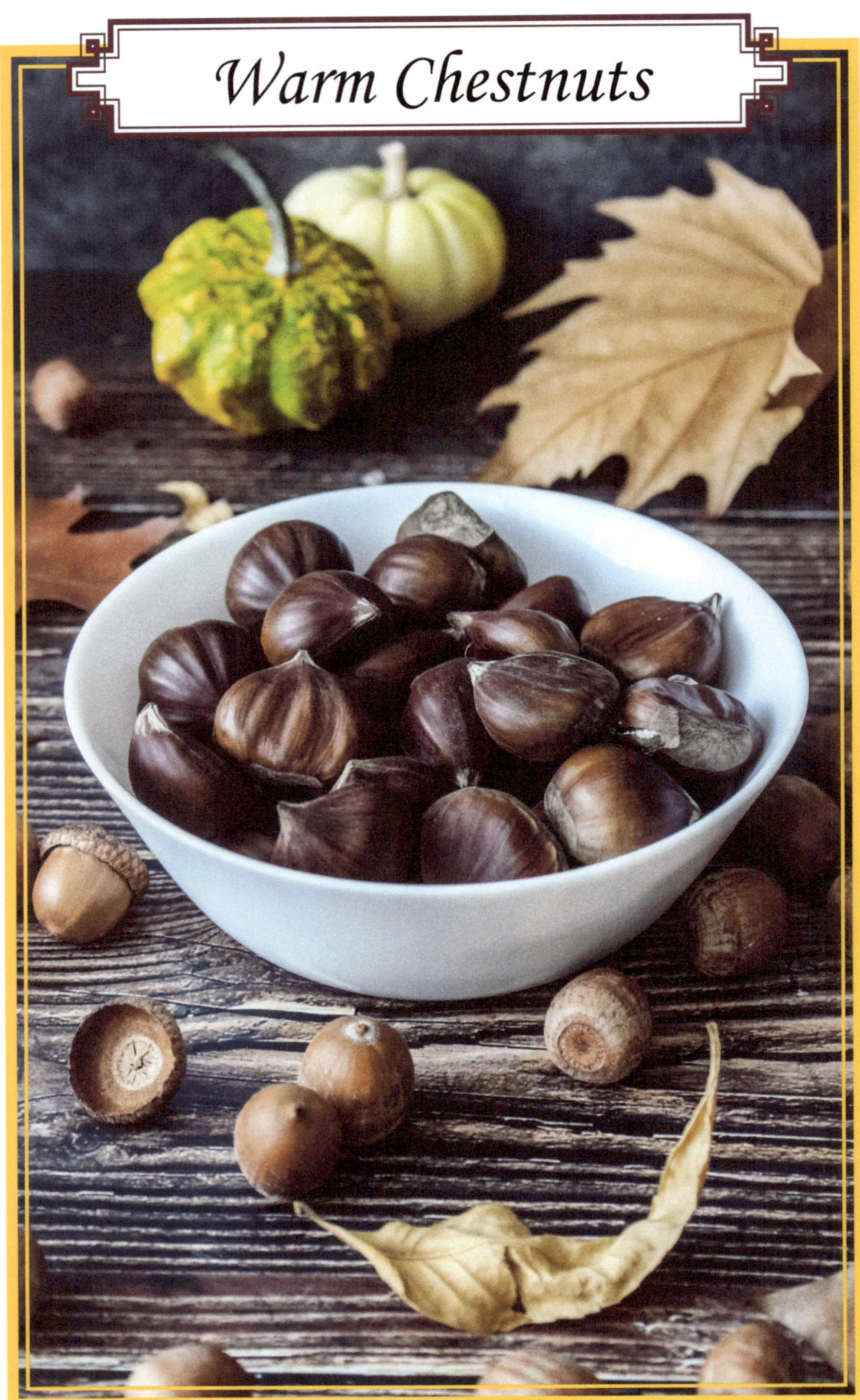

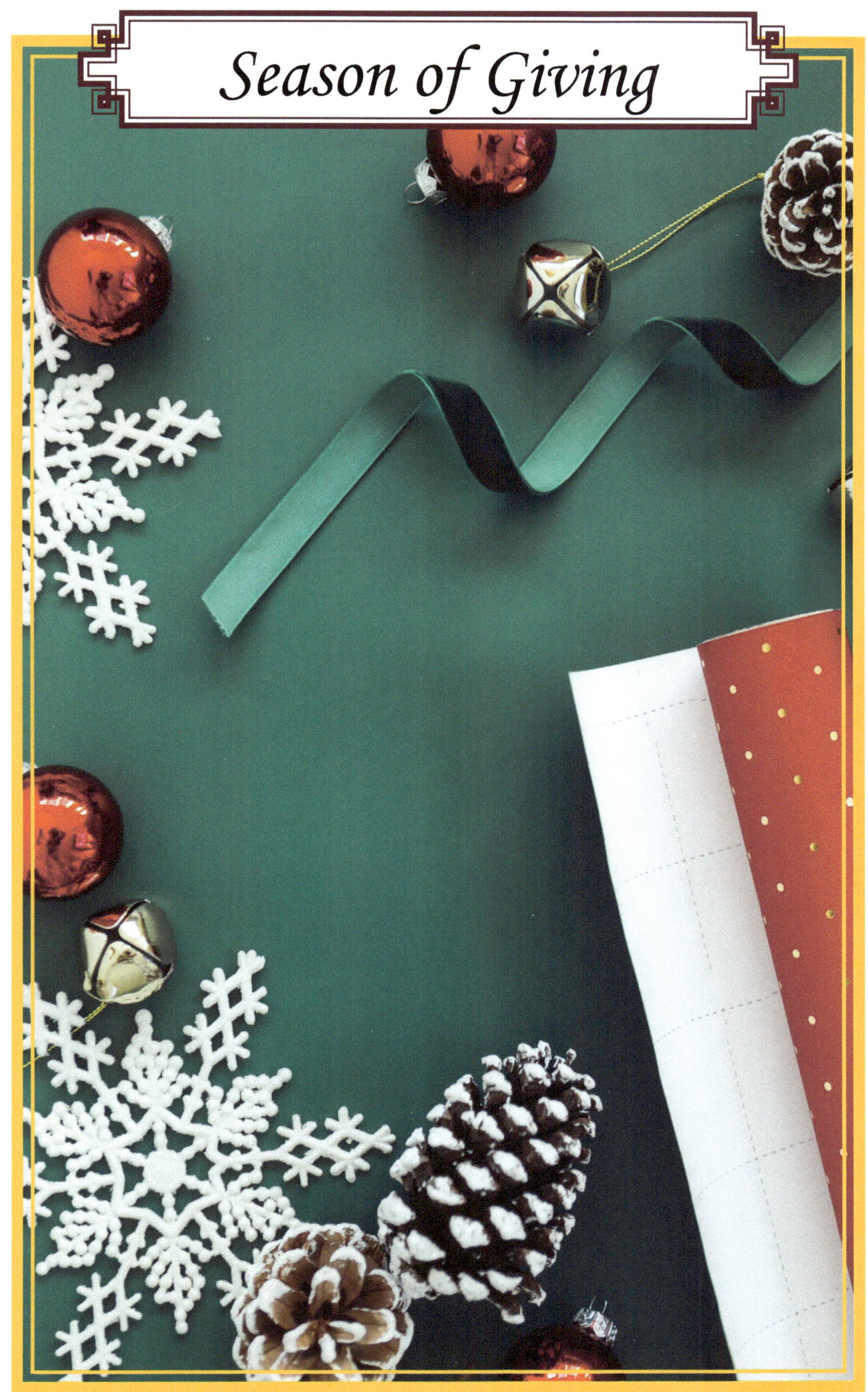
Season of Giving

Santa's Reindeer

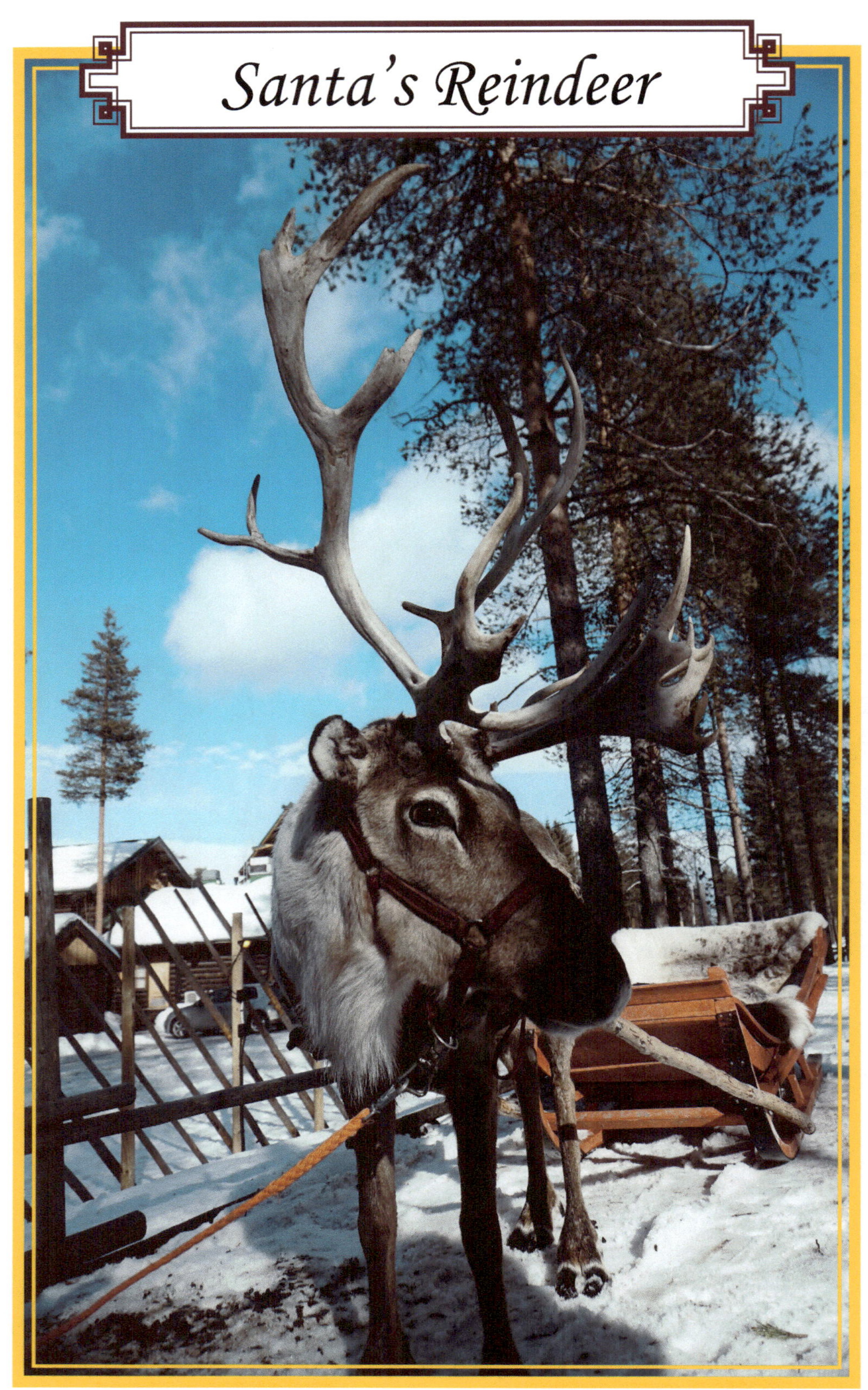

O Christmas Tree

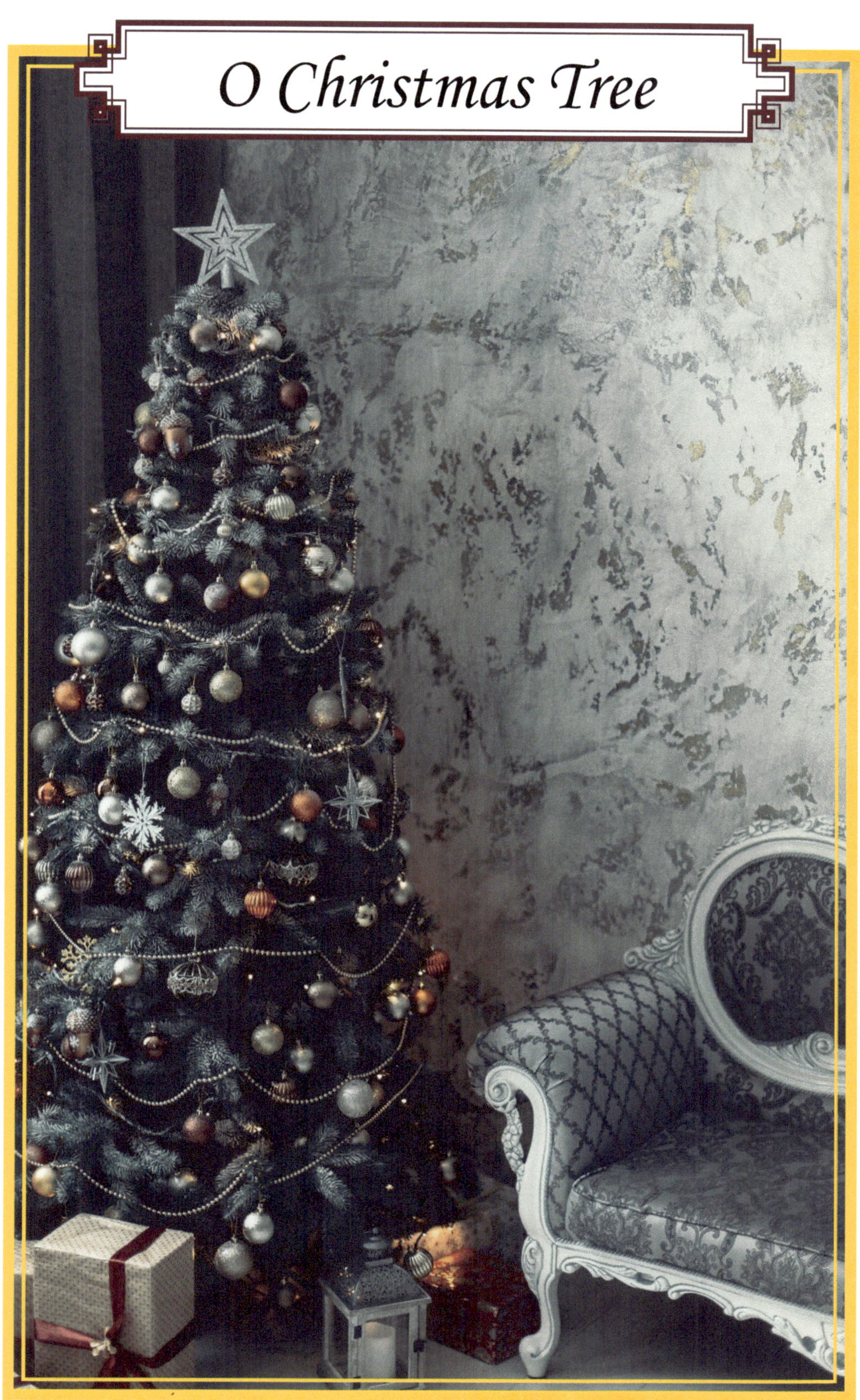

Stockings Were Hung

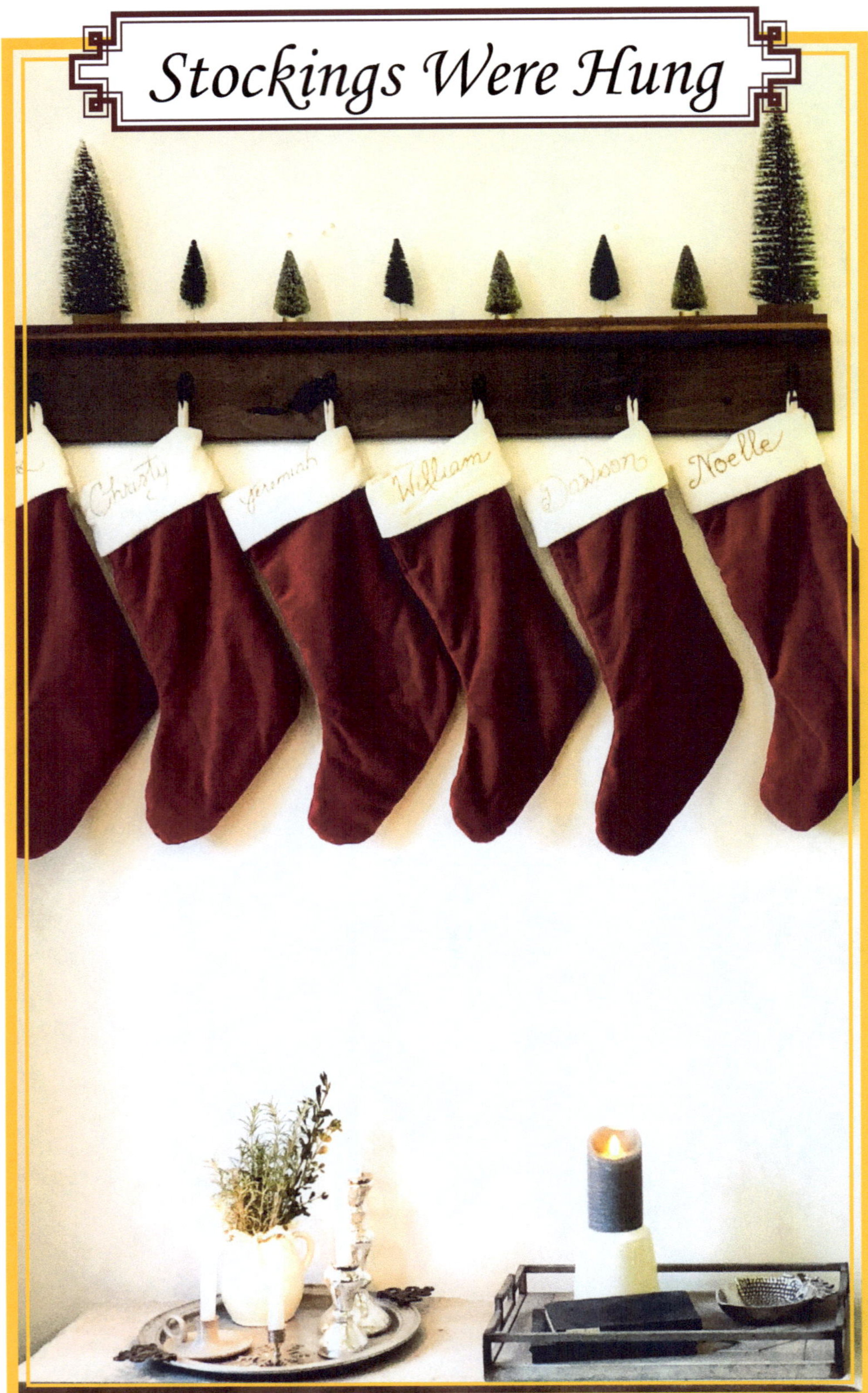

Gingerbread Men

Father Christmas

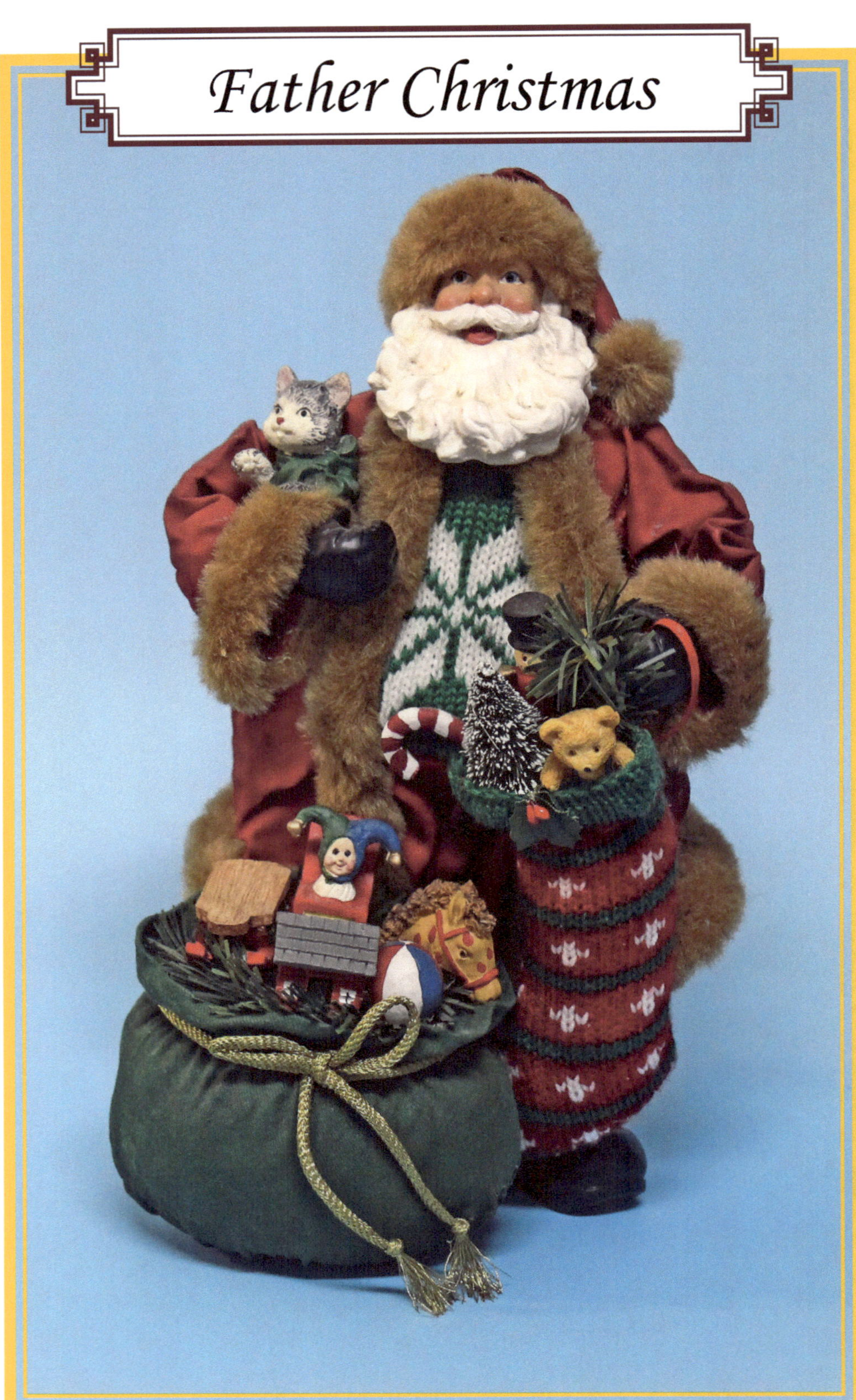

Gingerbread House

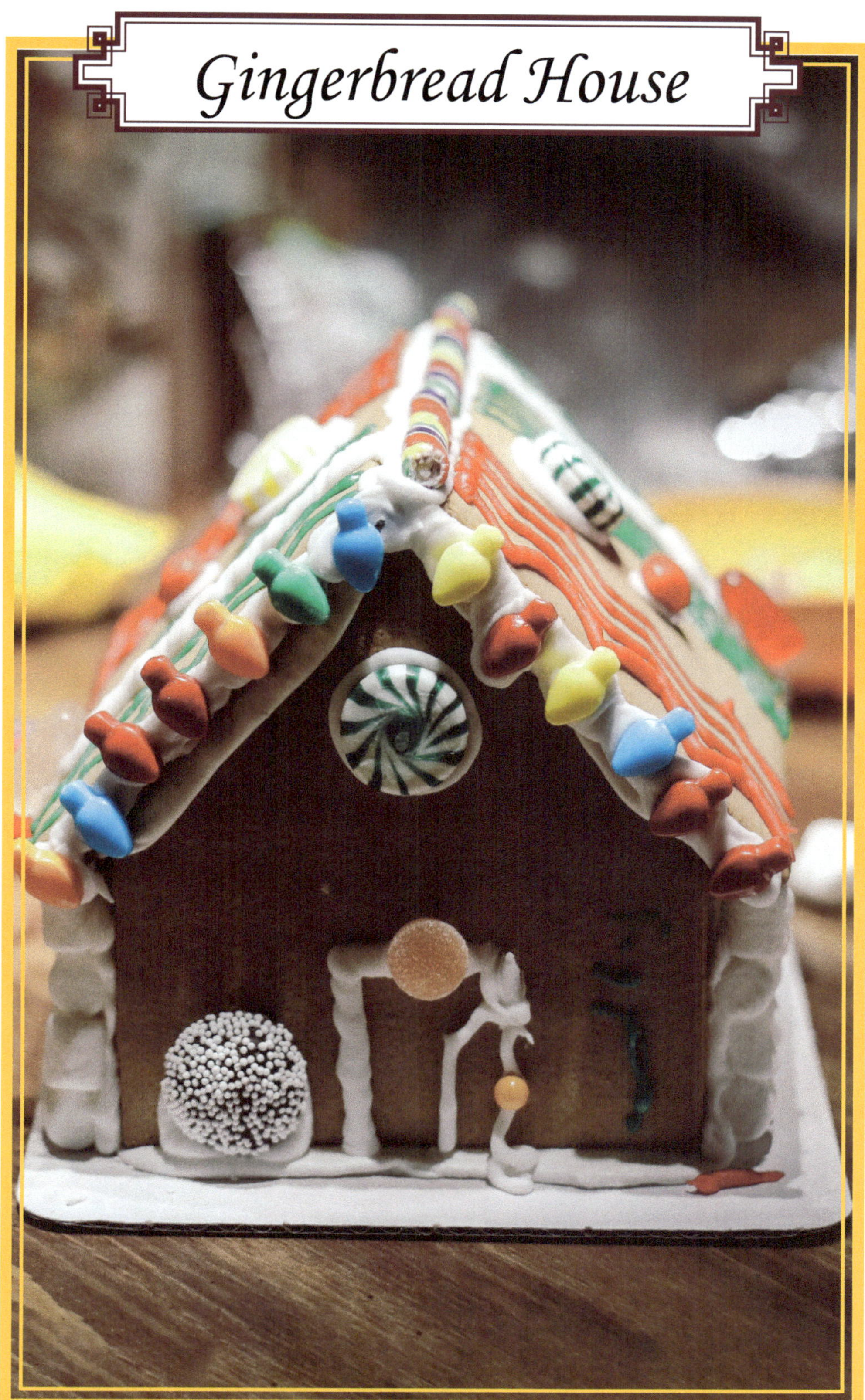

Laughter of Children

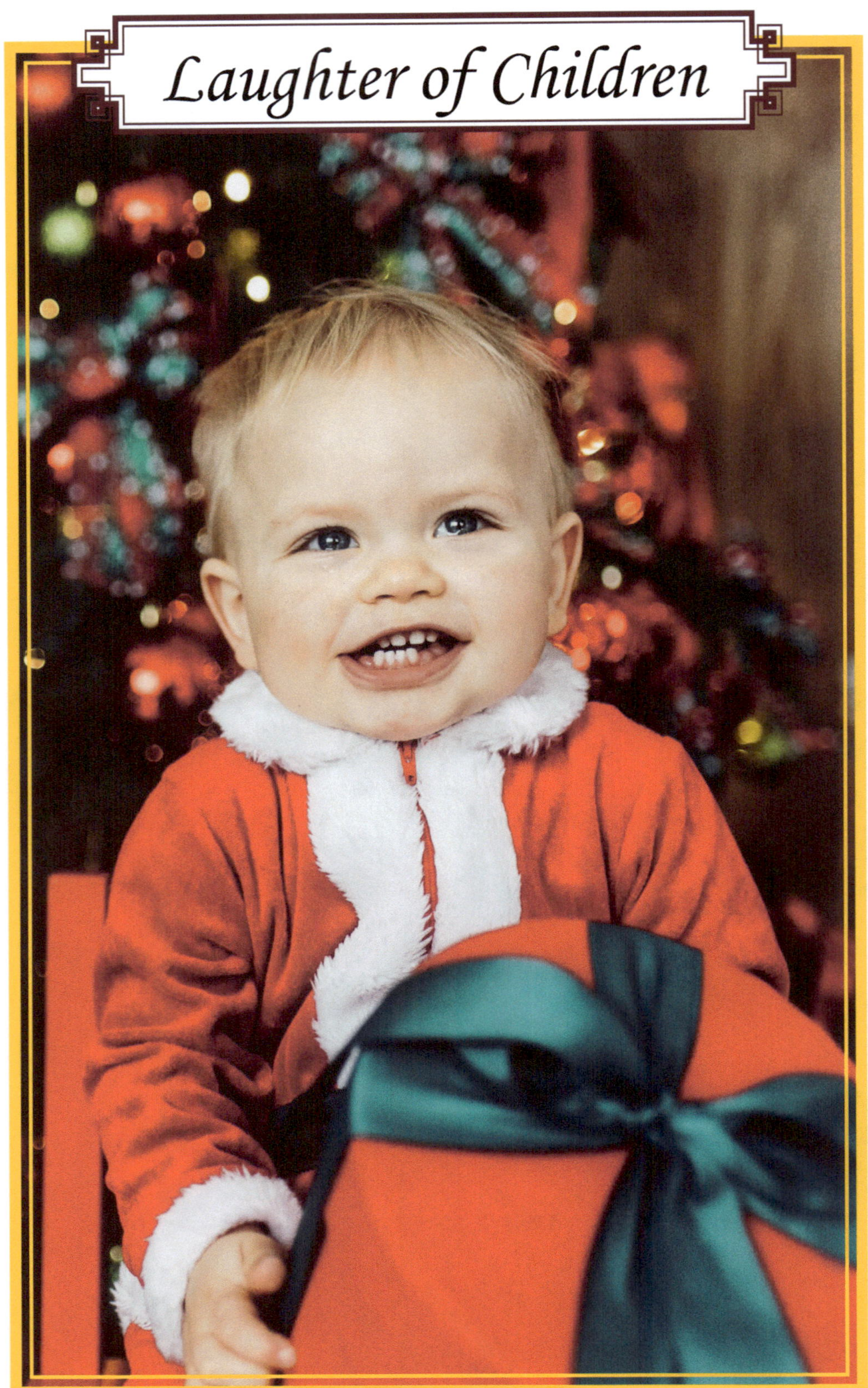

We Three Kings

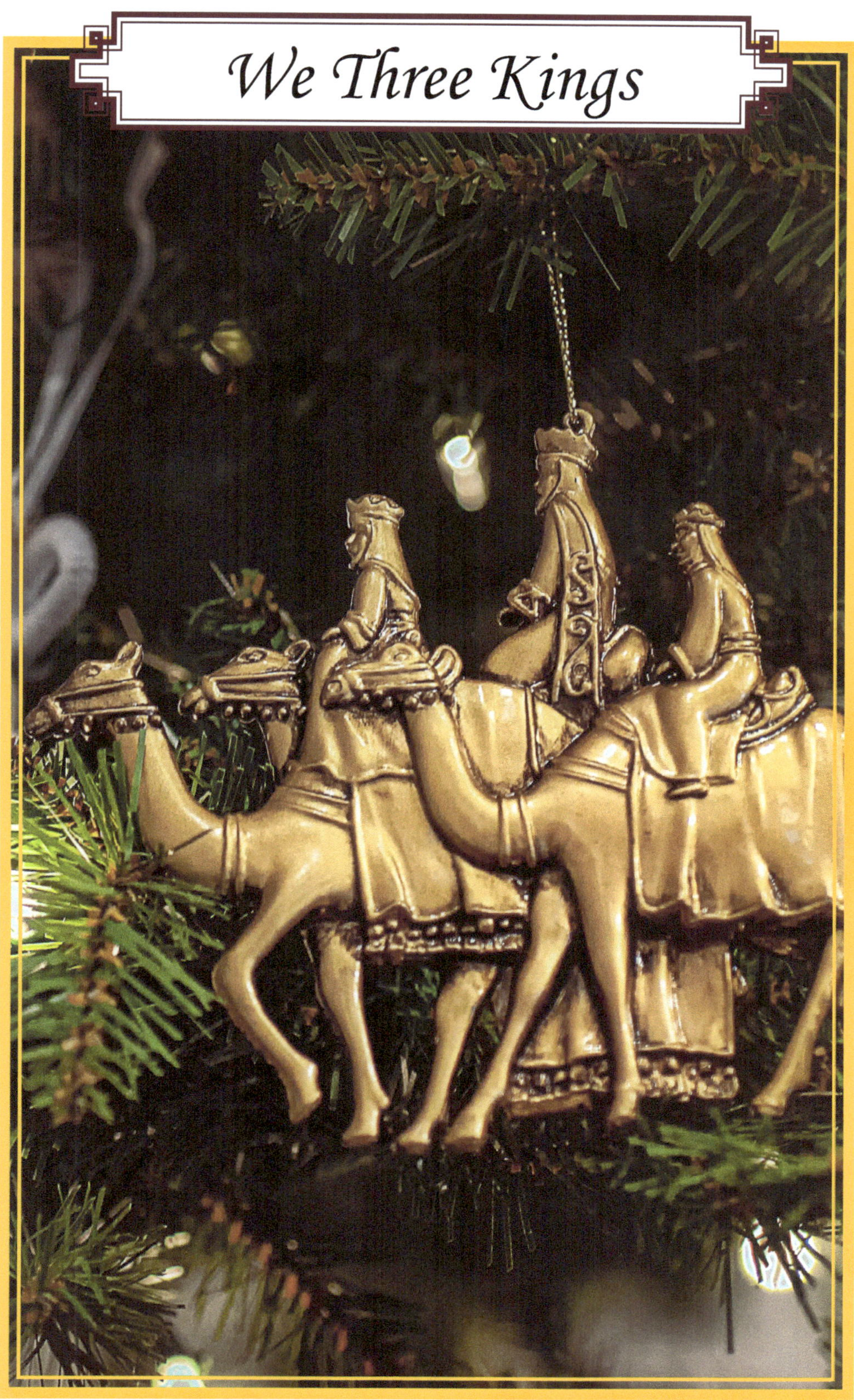